Gynaecology

T0075142

pocket tutor

JP

Gynaecology

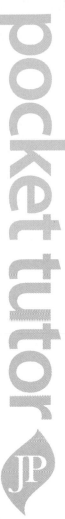

Jodi Keane BPhysio (Hons) MBBS (Hons) FRANZCOG
MIIA (Dist) CCPU
Consultant Obstetrician and Gynaecologist
Monash Health
Assessment Coordinator (Women's Health)
Monash University
Victoria, Australia

Manda Raz MBBS (Hons)
Resident Medical Officer
Monash Health
Victoria, Australia

Shavi Fernando MBBS (Hons) BMedSc (Hons)
FRANZCOG PhD
Consultant Obstetrician and Gynaecologist
Monash Health
Director of Undergraduate Curriculum
(Women's Health)
School of Clinical Sciences
Curriculum and Assessment Lead (Women's Health)
Monash University
Victoria, Australia

JP
medical
publishers

© 2022 Jaypee Brothers Medical Publishers

Published by Jaypee Brothers Medical Publishers,
4838/24 Ansari Road, New Delhi, India

Tel: +91 (011) 43574357   Fax: +91 (011)43574390

Email: info@jpmedpub.com, jaypee@jaypeebrothers.com
Web: www.jpmedpub.com, www.jaypeebrothers.com

JPM is the imprint of Jaypee Brothers Medical Publishers.

The rights of Jodi Keane, Manda Raz and Shavi Fernando to be identified as the authors of this work have been asserted by them in accordance with the Copyright, Designs and Patents Act 1988.

ISBN: 978-1-78779-123-7

British Library Cataloguing in Publication Data
A catalogue record for this book is available from the British Library

Library of Congress Cataloging in Publication Data
A catalog record for this book is available from the Library of Congress

Development Editor:	Harsha Madan
Editorial Assistant:	Keshav Kumar
Cover Design:	Seema Dogra

Preface

It is an undisputed fact that half of the population are female.

It is also hard to dispute that prepubertal girls, adolescents, adult cycling women, pre- and post-menopausal women all have gynaecological needs.

These needs are not always well met. Furthermore, the common clinical presentations, physiological underpinnings and management are often difficult to grasp, leading to poor understanding and fear in the junior clinician-fear of examining appropriately, fear of making the correct diagnosis and fear of managing relatively simple problems.

This leads to poorer outcomes.

Even in resource rich nations, women suffer the consequences of overly heavy menstruation, significant morbidity or mortality from unwanted or ectopic pregnancy and pain from treatable gynaecologic conditions that is diagnosed late or not at all. This needs to change.

Pocket Tutor Gynaecology provides an approachable, concise but comprehensive guide to the subject that is practical, straightforward and designed to give you, the clinician, pocket-sized access to confidence in appropriately assessing, diagnosing and treating common gynaecological presentations. It is intended for those who wish to include regular gynaecological care in their future practise but also for the general student and junior doctor who needs a refresh before a clinical encounter.

Clinical essentials and first principles chapters systematically outline key principles and anatomy and physiology, and the gynaecological lifespan is outlined in detailed chapters covering puberty, menstrual disorders, reproduction, and the menopause transition. There are also dedicated chapters covering common consequences of genital diseases, as well as childbearing, prolapse and incontinence and of gynaecological cancers.

Throughout the book we have included practical tips, useful diagrams and clinical images, examination techniques and tips as well as management options and their theoretical underpinnings to aid the junior clinician. We also emphasise woman-centred and sensitive clinical care.

We hope *Pocket Tutor Gynaecology* provides you with a solid grounding on your journey in the field of gynaecology, regardless of your final destination. Whether you are a medical student or a junior doctor, *Pocket Tutor Gynaecology* is your portable guide to understanding concepts, passing exams and providing clinical care during your gynaecology term.

Jodi Keane
Shavi Fernando
Manda Raz
November 2021

Contents

Acknowledgements

Yet again I find myself grateful to work with passionate and skilled co-authors on a project, this has made a mountain of a task a remarkably feasible undertaking and one of which we are all very proud. My family continue to grow, thrive and these days prefer electronic devices to children's television. Lily, Gemma and Rosie, thank you for your patience with an old-fashioned book. Sir Chas remains the best Sir I know from a field of one and absolutely a knight in shining school-run armour.

JK

Thanks to my co-authors, mentors, colleagues and patients, who continue to inspire me to pursue excellence.

MR

Thanks to my co-authors for their hard work and persistence. Thanks to my wife Sharmayne and children, Ellara and Arlen, who have allowed me extra time on top of a busy schedule to complete this book.

SF

First principles

1.1 Introduction

A thorough understanding of pelvic anatomy and normal physiological transitions during the reproductive phase is required to be able to competently care for girls and women throughout their lifespan.

This chapter outlines basic knowledge of gynaecological anatomy and the reproductive cycle that you will require as a foundation for further knowledge.

1.2 Normal (embryological) development of the genital tract

Key events

The development of the female genital tract has three key embryologic events. These are the differentiation of the gonad into an ovary, female differentiation of internal genital organs and female differentiation of external genital organs (**Figure 1.1**).

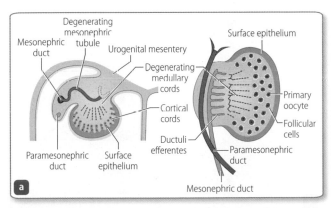

Figure 1.1 Female genital tract development. (a) Development of the ovaries; (b) Development of internal genitalia and (c) Development of external genitalia. *Continues overleaf*

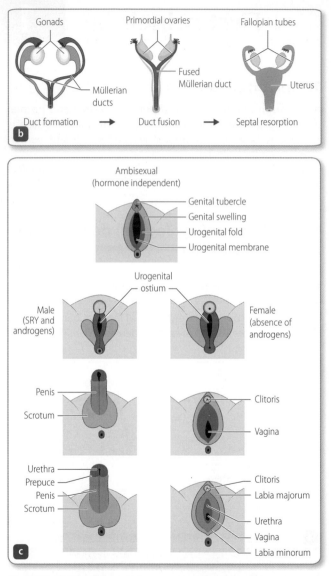

Figure 1.1 *Continued*

The embryologic gonad forms an ovary in the female fetus and a testicle in the male fetus. The testicle produces Müllerian-inhibiting substance (MIS), which inhibits the development of female internal genitalia in males (see below).

The ovary does not produce MIS. The fetal ovary also forms all primordial ova that the female will have throughout her future lifespan. New oocytes are not created past this point.

The internal genital organs are pluripotent in early fetal development and contain the Müllerian ducts and Wolffian ducts, both of which are closely associated with the embryonic kidney. The Müllerian ducts can develop into female internal genitalia (fallopian tubes, uterus, cervix and upper vagina), while the Wolffian ducts can develop into male internal genitalia.

The external genital organs include the labia majora, labia minora, clitoris and lower vagina. These have precursor structures (genital tubercle and labioscrotal folds) that respond to either fetal oestrogen or testosterone to differentiate into female or male external genital organs, respectively.

Developmental sequence

Both internal and external genital organ development is guided by sex steroid production from the gonad together with the presence or absence of MIS.

Internal genitalia

In a normal female fetus, the absence of testosterone and MIS causes the Wolffian ducts to regress and the Müllerian ducts to fuse in the mid-line, forming the upper vagina, cervix and uterus. The uppermost parts do not normally fuse and remain separate on either side of the uterus as the fallopian tubes (**Figure 1.2**). The lowermost part fuses with the developing lower vagina from the external genital organs and the vagina is canalised (opened) (**Figure 1.3**).

This principle of mid-line fusion, followed by vertical fusion with the developing external genitalia, is fundamental to understanding normal internal genital anatomy and how errors in this process can lead to failure of development of one side, failure of

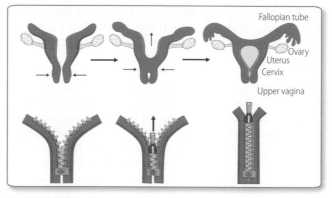

Figure 1.2 Mid-line fusion.

Guiding principle

Abnormalities of the Müllerian ducts are common and include bilateral agenesis [Mayer–Rokitansky–Küster–Hauser (MRKH) syndrome], unilateral agenesis or hypogenesis (unicornuate uterus or rudimentary horn), abnormalities of mid-line fusion (didelphys, septum or arcuate uterus) and abnormalities of vertical fusion with the external genitalia (cloacal defect and transverse vaginal septum) (**Figure 1.4**).

Pelvic ultrasound will identify most Müllerian malformations and should always include views of the kidneys. Because of the developmental proximity to the mesonephric ducts and the fetal kidney, mal-development of the Müllerian system is associated with abnormalities of the renal tract.

mid-line fusion for all or part of the Müllerian duct and failure of vertical fusion with the external genital organs with anatomical obstruction. It is also possible for the lower genital tract to erroneously connect with the alimentary tract and form a common exit termed the 'cloaca'.

External genitalia

The external genitalia develop from the fetal genital tubercle and labioscrotal folds. Oestrogen results in the urethra remaining posterior to the developing clitoris and not running through the genital tubercle, as it differentiates (as occurs in a male fetus). Similarly, the labioscrotal folds do not meet in the mid-line and form labia, which meet posterior to the developing vagina.

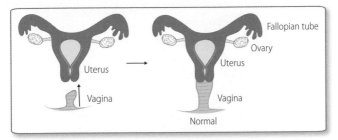

Figure 1.3 Vertical fusion.

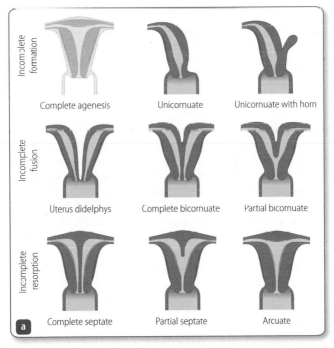

Figure 1.4 (a) Mid-line fusion problems and (b) Vertical fusion problems – transverse vaginal septum. *Continues overleaf*

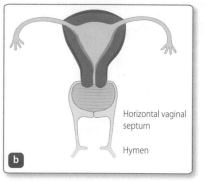

Figure 1.4 *Continued*

Horizontal vaginal
septum

Hymen

The lower vagina meets and fuses with the upper part of the vagina formed by the internal genitalia and the dividing tissue breaks down (canalises) to form a patent vaginal canal (**Figures 1.1** and **1.3**).

1.3 Pelvic anatomy

Bony pelvis

The pelvis comprises four bones: two innominate bones laterally and the sacrum and coccyx posteriorly. They are held together by strong ligaments and covered by muscle and fascia. Each innominate bone has three parts, which fuse together by puberty: (1) the wide ileum, located laterally; (2) the ischium, inferior, and the bone used to sit; and (3) the pubis, which meets the opposite side in the mid-line at the pubic ramus, the most anterior part of the bone (**Figure 1.5**).

The pelvic cavity is the space bounded by the bones of the pelvis. It is divided into the greater (false) and lesser (true) pelvises.

Lesser bony pelvis

The lesser pelvis, which contains the bladder and reproductive organs, is the part of the pelvic cavity between the pelvic inlet and the pelvic outlet (**Figure 1.6**).

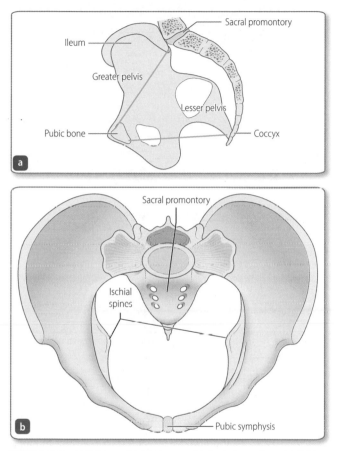

Figure 1.5 (a and b) Bony pelvis. The lesser pelvis lies between the pelvic inlet and the pelvic outlet. The greater pelvis is above the pelvic inlet.

The pelvic inlet is the aperture bordered by the superior margin of pubic symphysis (anteriorly), the arcuate line of each ileum (laterally) and the sacral promontory (posteriorly).

The pelvic outlet is the aperture bordered by the inferior margin of pubic symphysis (anteriorly), the inferior rami of pubis

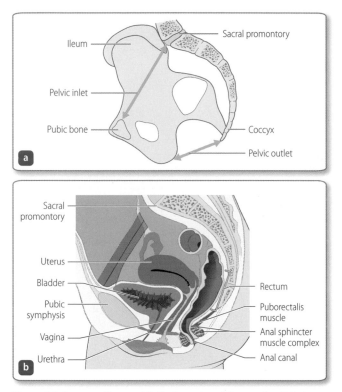

Figure 1.6 Contents of lesser pelvis. The internal genital organs lie within the pelvic inlet and outlet. The external genitalia lie below the outlet.

and ischial tuberosities (anterolaterally), the sacrotuberous ligaments (posterolaterally) and the tip of the coccyx (posteriorly).

The lesser pelvis is lined laterally by fascia over the pelvic bones, levator muscles of the pelvic floor and the muscles of the pelvic floor (below). Due to upright positioning and the challenges of expanding to accommodate birth of a fetus, this is the largest potential hernial portal in the body and disorders are common.

Greater bony pelvis

The bones of the greater pelvis, situated superior to the pelvic inlet, include the ilium and ala of sacrum. Mobile contents of the abdominal cavity including the small bowel and some large bowel sit within the greater pelvis. The greater pelvis is bounded by the abdominal wall anteriorly, the L5 or S1 vertebrae posteriorly and the iliac fossae posterolaterally.

Perineum and pelvic floor

The perineum lies inferior to the pelvis (and pelvic floor) and refers to the surface area of the body which sits on a bicycle seat. It is bounded by the symphysis pubis anteriorly; the inferior pubic rami, inferior ischial rami and sacrotuberous ligaments laterally; and the coccyx posteriorly. The anterior half contains the external genitalia and the posterior half contains the anus.

Separating the perineum and the pelvis is a muscular and ligamentous diaphragm known as the pelvic floor, which is traversed by the urethra, vagina and rectum (**Figure 1.7**). The principal muscle forming the pelvic floor is the levator ani. This thin, yet strong, muscle helps to support the pelvic viscera and is innervated by the pudendal nerve.

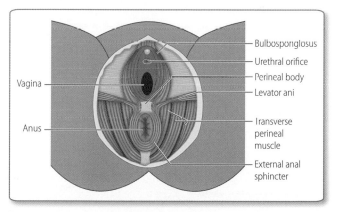

Vagina

Anus

Bulbospongiosus
Urethral orifice
Perineal body
Levator ani
Transverse perineal muscle
External anal sphincter

Figure 1.7 Pelvic floor and perineal muscles.

The perineum is divided by an imaginary line passing through the ischial tuberosities into a urogenital triangle anteriorly and an anal triangle posteriorly (**Figure 1.8**).

Pelvic muscles, nerves and vasculature
Muscles
The pelvic bones provide attachment for major muscle groups involved in movement of the lower limb (e.g. psoas, iliacus, rectus femoris, sartorius, adductors, gluteals, piriformis), spine and trunk (e.g. rectus abdominis, erector spinae, quadratus lumborum, external and internal oblique muscles) and pelvic floor (above).

The muscles of the pelvic floor are more relevant to gynaecology, as they are damaged in parturition and relevant in gynaecological repair.

Nerves
The nerves of the pelvis can be divided into somatic (under voluntary control) and autonomic (involuntary – sympathetic and parasympathetic function) as well as those which supply

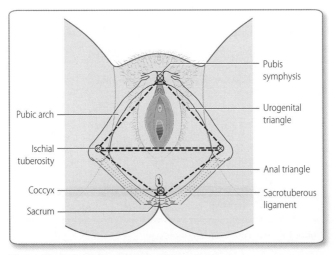

Figure 1.8 Genital and anal triangles of the perineum.

the organs and tissue of the pelvis and those that pass through to innervate the lower limb.

Somatic nerves include the pudendal nerve. Autonomic nerves carry sympathetic supply via the hypogastric and sacral nerves and parasympathetic supply via the pelvic nerve.

These nerves are important to gynaecologists, as they may be injured by gynaecologic procedures and parturition (childbirth).

Nerve injury This is graded by severity into neuropraxia, axonotmesis and neurotmesis, meaning compression with conduction disruption, division of the axons and division of the entire nerve in order of increasing severity. Neuropraxia recovers spontaneously with remyelination as does axonotmesis although this takes longer. Neurotmesis requires surgical repair to achieve any recovery of function and this is usually incomplete. Most gynaecologic injuries are neuropraxias and axonotmesis.

Nerve plexuses to lower limb Many major plexuses and lower limb peripheral nerves also pass to the lower limb via the pelvis. These include the lumbosacral plexus formed from the dorsal rami of nerve roots L1-S3 with a small contribution from T12 and its main branches, the sciatic nerve, femoral nerve and obturator nerve. This plexus lies within the psoas muscle and its branches arise from this muscle and arc through the pelvic sidewalls and out through sacral foramina and under the inguinal ligament into the anterior, medial and posterior lower limb (**Figure 1.9**).

Branches of the lumbosacral plexus with relevance of gynaecology and their significance are tabulated in **Table 1.1**.

Intrinsic pelvic somatic nerves The most important intrinsic nerve of the pelvis is the pudendal nerve. This arises from the sacral component of the lumbosacral plexus and has sensory supply of the external genitalia, clitoris, perineum, perianal skin and motor supply to the external urethral (voluntary) sphincter and external anal (voluntary) sphincter.

It is damaged in parturition and this damage can be permanent with stretch and ischaemic injury caused by prolonged

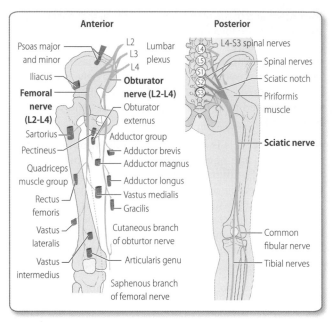

Figure 1.9 Limb nerve plexus traversing the pelvis.
Note:
Femoral nerve (L2-L4): Exists pelvis under inguinal ligament anteriorly. Innervates hip flexors and knee extensors
Obturator nerve (L2-L4): Exists pelvis through obturator foramen. Innervates muscles of medial thigh
Sciatic nerve (L4-S3): Exists pelvis through greater sciatic foramen posteriorly. Innervates posterior thigh and muscles of leg and foot

compression by a fetal head in second stage leading to loss of perineal sensation, sexual sensation and urinary and faecal incontinence.

Autonomic pelvic nerves The autonomic nervous supply includes sympathetic and parasympathetic innervation. The sympathetic supply of the body is carried along the sides of the vertebral canal as a sympathetic plexus whereas the parasympathetic supply exits at two sites, cranially as the vagus nerve

Nerve	Supply	Relevance
Lateral cutaneous nerve of thigh	Skin on lateral thigh	Can be compressed with blade of retractor during laparotomy
• Iliohypogastric • Ilioinguinal	• Supra-pubic skin sensation • Medial thigh and parts of external genitalia sensation • Both: Motor to lower transversus abdominis and internal oblique muscles	• Can be injured during laparotomy by compression with retractor or cut with lateral extension of Pfannenstiel incision • Both nerves pass within external/internal oblique muscle and are vulnerable to stretch or transection when these muscles are stretched or cut for access
Genitofemoral	Upper medial thigh, labia majora and mons pubis sensation	Can be injured during groin node dissection
Femoral nerve	• Motor to some hip flexors and medial rotators and knee extensors • Sensory to anteromedial thigh, medial foot and leg (via saphenous branch)	• Injured by stretch with excessive hip extension/knee flexion during laparoscopy – weakness of hip flexion, knee extension and numbness in sensory distribution • Can also be compressed by deep retractor blade during hysterectomy
Obturator nerve	• Motor to adductors of thigh • Sensory to medial thigh	• Injured in pelvic lymph node dissection, if care is not taken to preserve the nerve, which runs through the middle of the lymph node complex • Also injured with transobturator tape procedures for urinary incontinence

Table 1.1 Branches of the lumbosacral plexus relevant to gynaecology.

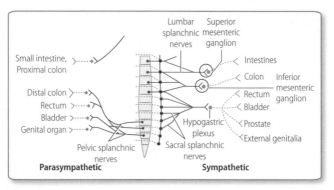

Figure 1.10 Autonomic pelvic nerves.

Source: Gest TR. (2000). Learning Modules – Medical Gross Anatomy: Introduction to Autonomics. [online] Available from https://anatomy.elpaso.ttuhsc.edu/modules/intro_autonomics_2_module/autonomics_12.html. [Last accessed from August, 2021].

Clinical insight

A small cervical biopsy is well tolerated, as the cervix has visceral but not somatic innervation. Pain is therefore perceived as pelvic, aching and not sharp, despite sharp excision with biopsy forceps. This means that local anaesthesia is rarely required. This is also the reason that cervical dilatation with intra-uterine device (IUD) insertion can cause hypotension and shock (vasovagal), as the cervix is innervated via the parasympathetic pelvic nerve.

and sacrally as the pelvic nerve (called craniosacral outflow) (**Figure 1.10**).

Sympathetic innervation is responsible for inhibition of defecation and urination. Parasympathetic innervation is responsible for facilitation of these processes. Parasympathetic innervation controls genital arousal changes and orgasm.

The autonomic pelvic nerves include the hypogastric nerve, the sacral and the pelvic splanchnic nerves. They form the inferior hypogastric plexus deep to the peritoneum in the pre-sacral space and supply sympathetic and parasympathetic innervation to the distal rectum, bladder and genital organs, notably including the cervix, which feels visceral pain via fibres carried in the pelvic nerve.

Sympathetic fibres are carried in the sacral splanchnic nerves from the sympathetic trunk and parasympathetic fibres arise from S2-S4 and are carried in the pelvic nerve.

Anterior abdominal wall anatomy

The anterior abdominal wall is composed of muscles, nerves, vessels and fascia. It is the site of common incisions for laparoscopy and open surgery, and connects to the pelvic bones. A knowledge of anatomy of the anterior abdominal wall is required to perform safe pelvic surgery.

Muscles

The major muscles forming the anterior abdominal wall are grouped into mid-line and lateral muscles.

Mid-line muscles These are the rectus abdominis and pyramidalis muscles. Together, they make up over half the anterior abdominal wall.

The rectus abdominis muscle extends from the lower costal cartilages superiorly to the pubic crest inferiorly. It is anchored transversely by attachment to the anterior layer of the rectus fascia at tendinous intersections. These fibrous bands give rise to the so-called 'six-pack' appearance of the tensed rectus abdominis. The rectus fascia ends at the anatomical landmark known as the arcuate line, where there is a change in arrangement of the layers forming the anterior abdominal wall; this means that incisions made for a caesarean section do not encounter the posterior rectus sheath because it does not exist below the umbilicus (**Figure 1.11**).

The pyramidalis muscle, which is absent in 20% of people, is anterior to the inferior part of the rectus abdominis and attaches to the anterior pubis. The pyramidalis muscle ends in and tenses the linea alba, the thick mid-line formed by fusion of the two bilateral aponeuroses of the abdominal muscles. The linea alba is wide superior to the umbilicus and then tapers inferior to it.

Lateral muscles These are the external oblique, internal oblique and transverse abdominis muscles. Their fleshy bodies

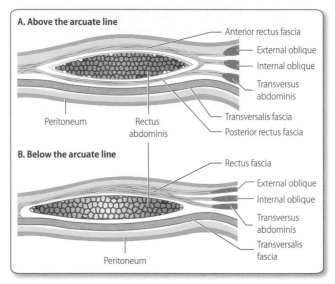

Figure 1.11 Anterior abdominal wall.

become aponeurotic, as they approach the lateral border of the rectus abdominis muscle. These muscles also contribute to the structure of the inguinal ligament.

Nerves

Innervation of the anterior abdominal wall derives from the T7 down to the L1 nerve roots. T7-L1 spinal nerves travel inferiorly and medially giving rise to lateral and anterior cutaneous nerves that traverse the fibres of the abdominal wall muscles to reach the skin.

Vessels

The anterior abdominal wall is supplied with blood from three sources:

1. Inter-costal and sub-costal arteries (direct branches of the aorta)

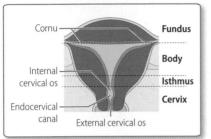

Figure 1.12 Uterine anatomy.

Cornu — **Fundus**

Body

Internal cervical os — **Isthmus**

Cervix

Endocervical canal —

External cervical os

2. Superior epigastric arteries (terminal branches of the internal thoracic artery)
3. Inferior epigastric arteries (terminal branches of the external iliac arteries)

Organs
The pelvis contains key organs in the genitourinary and gastrointestinal systems, as distal extensions for excretion as well as true intrinsic pelvic organs. The main organs of the pelvis are the uterus and fallopian tubes, ovaries and the bladder and rectum.

Uterus
Before pregnancy, the uterus measures 8 cm long. This increases to 38 cm by the time a normal pregnancy reaches term, at which stage the uterus lies just under the sternum. The uterus comprises a fundus, two lateral cornua, a body, an isthmus and a cervix (**Figure 1.12**).

Relations The relations of the uterus are:
- *Anteriorly*: The uterovesical pouch, separating it from the bladder and loops of the small intestine
- *Posteriorly*: The rectouterine pouch (of Douglas), separating it from the rectum
- *Laterally*: The fallopian tubes, ovaries, blood vessels and nerves, all embedded in the broad ligament; the ureters pass lateral to the uterus and inferior to the uterine vessels

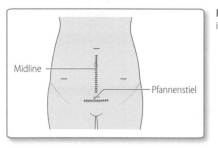

Figure 1.13 Common incisions.

The uterus receives blood predominantly from two large uterine arteries, which arise from the internal iliac arteries. The uterine arteries anastomose with terminal branches of the ovarian arteries (direct branches of the aorta).

Gynaecological surgical incisions
Pfannenstiel incision
This is a slightly curved horizontal incision made at the pubic hairline (**Figure 1.13**). A Joel–Cohen incision is slightly higher and horizontal. Both are frequently used. At the level of a routine Pfannenstiel incision, below the arcuate line of the rectus fascia, the following structures are encountered, from superficial to deep:
- Skin
- Superficial fatty (Camper's) fascia
- Superficial membranous (Scarpa's) fascia
- Rectus fascia (the rectus sheath) enclosing the rectus abdominis muscle
- Pre-peritoneal fat and parietal peritoneum
- The bladder (if it is not empty)

Mid-line Incision
This incision is made through the linea alba. It is a clean and rapid way to access the abdomen because of the absence of blood vessels and nerves in the linea alba.

Mid-line incisions are usually made below the umbilicus; however, when wide abdominal access is required, they are extended above the umbilicus. This is rare in benign gynaecology, but common in cancer surgery.

Laparoscopy incision

This is a keyhole incision made to insert a camera or laparoscopic surgical tool into the abdomen, particularly for gynaecological operations. Common laparoscopic incision sites are umbilical, supra-pubic and lateral abdominal.

Care is needed to avoid damaging peripheral nerves and vessels that cross the area of incision or insertion. In particular, this applies to the inferior epigastric vessels with lateral port sites – these should be visualised using the primary entry laparoscope and the planned lateral port entries made away from their path on the internal surface of the anterior abdominal wall. They are visible as pulsatile structures through the parietal peritoneum.

The urinary bladder is also emptied to avoid injury with supra-pubic port insertion.

1.4 Normal menstrual cycle

Hypothalamic-pituitary-ovarian axis

The hypothalamic-pituitary-ovarian (HPO) axis involves each of these organs, which act together to produce reproductive hormones, initiate puberty and regulate the menstrual cycle.

The arcuate nucleus of the hypothalamus secretes pulsatile gonadotropin-releasing hormone (GnRH), which travels in the portal circulation to the anterior pituitary gland. Here, it stimulates the release of follicle-stimulating hormone (FSH) and luteinising hormone (LH). These then act directly on the ovary to produce oestrogen and progesterone (**Figure 1.14**).

Throughout most of the menstrual cycle, oestrogen and progesterone provide negative feedback on the pituitary gland and hypothalamus, reducing GnRH secretion and reducing the release of FSH and LH. At low levels of oestrogen, LH secretion from the pituitary gland is suppressed but at higher concentrations of oestrogen, LH secretion is stimulated. Therefore, once

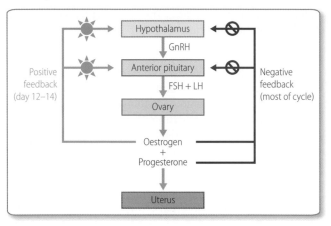

Figure 1.14 The HPO axis.
(FSH, follicle-stimulating hormone; GnRH, gonadotropin-releasing hormone; HPO, hypothalamic-pituitary-ovarian; LH, luteinising hormone)

Clinical insight

Variation in the length of the follicular phase is most responsible for variations in overall cycle length, as luteal phase duration is relatively constant at 14 days. In other words, in a woman with a 35-day cycle, her follicular phase lasts approximately at 21 days, as her luteal phase is constant at 14 days.

a dominant follicle develops and starts to produce more oestrogen (see *ovulatory cycle* below), an LH 'surge' is triggered, which ultimately results in ovulation.

Ovarian cycle

The number of oocytes that a female possesses rapidly declines throughout development. At 20 weeks of gestation, a female human fetus contains 6–7 million oocytes. At birth, she has 1–2 million oocytes and by puberty, 300,000 oocytes. Of these, only 400–500 oocytes will actually reach the stage of ovulation. Menopause occurs when the effective ovarian oocyte supply is depleted, with menopausal ovaries containing mostly dense stroma with interspersed rare oocytes. Unlike sperm, new oocytes cannot be created.

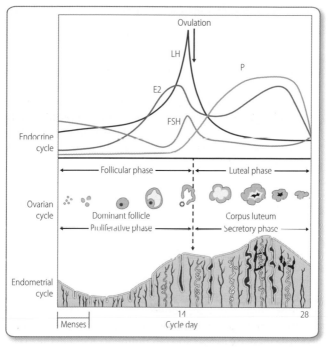

Figure 1.15 Ovarian and endometrial cycles.

The ovarian cycle is divided into two phases (**Figure 1.15**). The follicular phase (from menstruation to ovulation), which lasts for 10–14 days and the luteal phase (from ovulation to menses), which lasts for 14 days.

Follicular phase

At the beginning of the menstrual cycle, ovarian hormones (oestrogen and progesterone) are low. Following the demise of the corpus luteum, the withdrawal of progesterone negative feedback results in an increase in FSH. This results in the recruitment of ovarian follicles, with each follicle producing some oestrogen, which in turn causes endometrial proliferation.

As the growing follicles produce inhibin B and more oestrogen negative feedback is exerted on the pituitary gland. This causes a reduction in FSH by the mid-point of the follicular phase. One follicle becomes dominant and grows further, smaller follicles are not able to survive low FSH and stop growing. As the oestrogen concentration progressively increases towards the end of the follicular phase, positive feedback starts and an LH 'surge' occurs, triggering ovulation 24–36 hours later.

Luteal phase

At ovulation, oestrogen decreases. The remaining cells from the ruptured follicle form the corpus luteum, which secretes oestrogen, inhibin A and mostly progesterone. Progesterone increases significantly after ovulation. The increase in pro-gesterone, oestrogen and inhibin A result in a decline in FSH and LH (negative feedback). In the absence of fertilisation, the corpus luteum demises after 14 days, causing a decline in progesterone and oestrogen. This removes the negative feedback on the hypothalamus and pituitary gland, result-ing in an increase in FSH and re-commencement of the cycle.

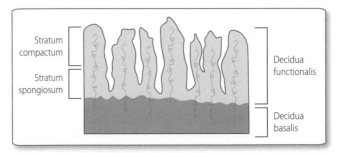

Figure 1.16 Endometrium layers.

Endometrial cycle

Occurring concurrently with the ovarian cycle, the endometrium is prepared to receive a fertilised oocyte (zygote). In the absence of implantation, menstruation occurs. This is the endometrial cycle.

The endometrium is composed of layers (**Figure 1.16**). The most superficial layer is the decidua functionalis, which comprises the most superficial two-thirds of the endometrium. This layer is very responsive to reproductive hormones and is the part of the endometrium that sheds with menses. It is comprised of the stratum spongiosum (deep layer) and the stratum compactum (superficial layer).

Deep to the decidua functionalis is the decidua basalis. This is the source of endometrial regeneration after menses. This layer has no significant monthly proliferation and is relatively unresponsive to hormones.

The endometrial cycle is divided into two phases that coincide with the phases of the ovarian cycle (**Figure 1.15**).

The proliferative phase begins after the onset of menses on day 1 of the cycle. Following this, the endometrium is approximately 1–2 mm thick. The increasing oestrogen released by the developing follicles results in mitotic proliferation of the decidua functionalis. The endometrial glands change from being straight, narrow and short into being long and tortuous glands preparing it for implantation. The cell type changes from low columnar into pseudo-stratified, with dense stroma containing minimal vascular structures. It is now ready for the secretory phase.

The secretory phase begins 48–72 hours following ovulation. The increased progesterone from the corpus luteum results in the secretion of protein-rich eosinophilic products from endometrial glands. There is a progressive decline in endometrial oestrogen receptor number, resulting in less proliferation. There is a shift to secretion from glycogen-containing glands on days 19–20 with maximal secretion occurring 6–7 days after ovulation. The endometrium is now ready for the blastocyst.

In the absence of implantation, the endometrial stroma remains unchanged until post-ovulatory day 7. At this point, endometrial spiral arteries lengthen and coil. At day 24, eosinophilia is visible in the peri-vascular stroma. Two days before menses, there is infiltration with polymorphs, which signals the onset of menses.

The demise of the corpus luteum results in a fall in oestrogen and progesterone as mentioned earlier. This causes spiral artery spasm and ischaemia of the endometrium. There is secretion of proteolytic enzymes, which further destroys the decidua functionalis. Secretion of prostaglandin F2α (PGF2α) results in vasoconstriction with further artery spasm and ischaemia as well as uterine contractions (cramps). Menstruation ensues.

Clinical essentials

2.1 Introduction

The gynaecological history and examination consist of a combination of general medical and surgical assessment together with a more specific and targeted gynaecological (and obstetric) appraisal.

A thorough history is important as it guides physical examination and these both, in turn, guide the selection of appropriate investigations. This then follows naturally into arriving at the correct diagnosis and planning optimal management and clinical care.

> ### Clinical insight
>
> The axiom 'history is 80% of the diagnosis' holds true in most of medicine including gynaecology and obstetrics and it is well worth perfecting this skill as you will be more clinically efficient, accurate and provide better care.

2.2 History

The principles of history taking in gynaecology are, in addition to standard medical and surgical history items, to capture coherently the spectrum of potential gynaecological complaints, assess well woman care including breast, cervical and other screening, discuss fertility control and plans and treat complications of natural events such as the menopause.

The sensitive nature of some gynaecological problems means they are not always disclosed. Both skill with discussing such matters, a tactful approach and attention to non-verbal cues are helpful in maximising your history taking. This should routinely include interviewing women in private to ensure they have the opportunity to discuss concerns freely, disclose past terminations or sexually transmitted infections and ensure they are safe from coercion, physical or sexual abuse. This can often be completed when examining under the guise of privacy without creating discord with the support person.

Building rapport

Building rapport with women is essential when history includes intimate items such as in gynaecology where routine enquiry regarding menstruation, sexual function, sexual pain, vaginal discharge and genital symptoms are routine.

Be guided by the woman's preference for a support person during her interview. Any partner or support person should be involved at the request of the woman and the woman is entitled to privacy from companions, if this is her preference. Be aware that in certain 'sensitive' situations, it may not be appropriate for the woman's intimate partner to attend (e.g. sexual assault). Rapport is achieved verbally and non-verbally.

- *Verbal rapport* is built by using the woman's name and repeating some of what she has said to indicate that you have been listening. This might include repeating the symptoms they described back to them.
- *Non-verbal* rapport refers to appropriate body language including handshaking, nodding and gesturing.

Allow adequate time for the woman to state her concerns, do not be afraid to listen as rarely will a woman talk for so long as to delay your consultation and time is often saved as the woman will feel her concerns have been acknowledged and this allows the history to move onto other elements without resistance.

Always explicitly state the history given is held in confidence unless the woman requests you disclose to another party with the exception of where legal reporting is mandatory.

Age

Age impacts significantly on formulating a differential diagnosis. Younger women, for example, are more likely to have menorrhagia (heavy periods) due to functional/hormonal issues and older women due to structural problems in the uterus such as fibroids or adenomyosis.

It also helps to inform what issues may be important for the woman. For example, a young teenager will be more interested in contraception than advice about infertility and a post-menopausal woman will not be interested in discussing contraception. Also, as age increases, issues around fertility become significant for women in their reproductive years.

Presenting problem

The presenting problem (or complaint) is the reason the woman seeks your help. It is a free statement usually given at the start of the consult. A common example is 'my periods are too heavy.'

This is always considered a symptom (i.e. not a diagnosis and not a clinical sign you identify on examination), which you will need to characterise to identify potential causes (differential diagnoses) by application of directed questions.

In order to facilitate a focussed and directed assessment of the patient, a detailed history of their presenting problem needs to be elicited. This will then allow a more detailed exploration of their symptoms and possible causes.

Gynaecological history

Menstrual history

Ask about the date of the first day of the last menstrual period (LMP).

Guiding principle

Symptoms, signs, investigations, diagnoses and differentials are not interchangeable terms. Using them correctly enhances the clarity of your clinical documentation and handover and gives an impression of competence.

A symptom is a problem the patient reports. A sign is a finding that you identify on examination and a diagnosis is the pathological cause of the symptom and/or sign after appropriate investigation.

Investigation is sometimes not required to make the diagnosis or may be minimal or extensive depending on the problem suspected (differential diagnosis).

Clinical insight

Questions that can be used to clarify their symptoms are (WWQQAAB):

- **W**hen (does the symptom present)?
- **W**here (is the symptom)?
- **Q**uality (of the symptom)?
- **Q**uantity (of the symptom)?
- **A**lleviating factors (does anything make the symptom improve)?
- **A**ggravating factors (does anything make the symptom worse)?
- **B**eliefs (what does the patient think her symptom is due to)?

The LMP is used to estimate which phase of their menstrual cycle in the woman is currently in (follicular/proliferative phase or luteal/secretory phase).

Also ask regarding the age of menarche (the age of their first period) and/or the age of menopause (if applicable). This can help to identify risk factors for some gynaecological conditions,

Clinical insight

There is a wide variety of 'normal.' Abnormality can only be established, if the patient is concerned or their life is affected by the variation – always treat the woman and not just the number.

Of course, if there is an associated major pathology, e.g. carcinoma, this is abnormal regardless of quality of life currently due to the health implications without treatment.

e.g. women who have early menarche and late menopause have a higher risk of endometrial carcinoma.

It is important to identify the characteristics of menstrual bleeding, in particular, regularity, heaviness and pain. A 'normal' menstrual cycle should be 28 days long and regular, with 3–5 days of bleeding in most cases. It should not be painful or heavy enough to affect day-to-day activities. In addition, there should not be any bleeding or pain between periods.

Regularity

Irregular periods are most commonly linked to polycystic ovarian syndrome, other causes uncommonly include thyroid disorders, benign pituitary tumours, adrenal gland dysfunction, and central (hypothalamic causes). The presence of an irregular cycle can also make it more difficult to conceive as a woman may not be ovulating regularly or at all.

Bleeding pattern and duration

Menstrual bleeding <2 days or >7 is defined as abnormal. The upper limit of normal blood loss is considered to be 80 mL.

However, as it is usually impracticable to measure the volume of menstrual loss, heavy bleeding is best regarded as bleeding the woman finds particularly inconvenient or associated with iron deficiency or anaemia.

Ask about other vaginal bleeding including inter-menstrual or post-coital bleeding, which can indicate cervical disease or endometrial pathology.

Excessive menstrual bleeding causes chronic anaemia, which should be treated with iron-rich diet and oral iron supplementation and the reason for the heavy menses corrected.

Cervical screening

Ask the woman if she is due for cervical screening.

This may be a Pap smear or human papillomavirus (HPV) deoxyribonucleic acid (DNA) test depending on the healthcare system.

Also enquire if she has ever had abnormal screening or treatment for cervical dysplasia in the past as this increases her chance of future problems.

It is useful to enquire regarding HPV vaccination as an automatic accompaniment as you are less likely to forget this item this way and can recommend vaccination in eligible women.

Contraception/hormonal treatments

Always ask regarding current contraception method, compliance, acceptability and side effects. It is important to also enquire about desires for future fertility, as this changes your treatment options and is an opportunity for preconception care, counselling and folate supplementation.

Contraceptive methods include non-hormonal, hormonal and barrier methods of contraception (refer to Chapter 6).

If the woman is peri-menopausal (has menopause symptoms but still some periods) or menopausal (has had no menstrual periods in 12 months in the absence of pregnancy or other pathology), also enquire regarding use of herbal, complementary and prescribed menopause hormonal therapy [hormone replacement therapy ('HRT')]. This may highlight other areas of their health that need addressing such as menopausal symptoms and is an opportunity for health education.

Sexual history

Enquire about previous episodes of sexually transmitted infections (STIs), pelvic inflammatory disease (PID) and their treatment.

Untreated or chronic STIs lead to adhesions and scarring of the fallopian tubes, uterine and pelvic cavity, contributing to ectopic pregnancy and chronic pain. Routinely offer screening for chlamydia and gonorrhoea to women <25 years old as STI is common in this population (estimated up to 5%).

Guiding principle

Learning new history items can be difficult and long lists commit poorly to memory. Mnemonics, by grouping bigger lists into smaller chunks, maximise your ability to retain complex lists efficiently and use them well.

Guiding principle

Any woman who has had major abdominal open surgery, in particular midline laparotomy, is at high risk of intra-peritoneal adhesions. This can increase the risk of damaging abdominal structures during any further surgery and changes both threshold for repeat surgery and technical factors around conduct.

As a part of the sexual history, it is important to identify if the woman is sexually active and in a safe and supportive relationship meaning not subject to emotional, financial, physical or sexual abuse. This line of questioning should occur without anyone else present in the consultation. Violence against women is more prevalent than many think and is an essential issue in the holistic management of women.

Medical history

Enquire about any condition requiring specialist input or active treatment. This includes any serious or severe respiratory, cardiac or renal disease as these alter your treatment options in many cases.

Surgical history

Enquire specifically about open and laparoscopic abdominal operations (e.g. bowel surgery, appendicectomy, cholecystectomy) and issues with general anaesthesia, such as allergies or intubation difficulties, due to morbid obesity or a narrow pharynx. These all also affect the best treatment option for the woman's presenting problem and allow you to assess safety of potential further surgery.

Medication history

In addition to recording regular medications, enquire specifically regarding:

- Analgesics, in particular opiate analgesia. Women with chronic pelvic pain often resort to opiate analgesia to manage their pain. This is not always appropriate as opiates do not treat pelvic pain effectively and are addictive. Chronic pelvic pain always needs to be managed in a multidisciplinary fashion involving chronic pain specialists, psychologists, gynaecologists and sometimes sexual health specialists

• Anticoagulants such as low-molecular-weight heparin or warfarin. These become relevant when considering menorrhagia as well as when planning operative intervention

• Antidepressants, including selective serotonin reuptake inhibitors. These may provide clues to a woman's mental state, but also may contribute to urinary dysfunction

Obstetric history
Enquire about all pregnancies including the number of terminations, miscarriages, ectopic pregnancies, live births and mode of delivery. This will help to inform further history taking and will highlight additional surgical history and fertility background (see Pocket Tutor Obstetrics).

Family history
Enquire regarding heritable gynaecological conditions. These include but are not limited to fibroids, infertility, recurrent miscarriage, gynaecological cancers and gynaecological surgery for benign indications.

Refer for genetic counselling if there is suspicion of a genetic condition which may increase the chance of familial cancers, e.g. BRCA mutation and ovarian cancer.

Social history
Living circumstances and finances have direct impact on the health of women. Drinking alcohol, smoking and illicit drug use are associated with mental health disorders, chronic pelvic pain and domestic violence.

Good practice point
Document each pregnancy in chronological location with year, place of birth, mode of birth, birthweight and complications. Generate a list of 'Gs and Ps', which are gravida (all pregnancies, regardless of outcome) and parity, all deliveries after 20 weeks' of gestation. Multiple pregnancies are denoted by a '+' and a stillbirth (after 20 weeks or birth weight <500 g) is denoted with a '−'.

Smoking also increases the risk of all gynaecological cancers.

Non-pharmacological methods (e.g. counselling and support group meetings), pharmacological agents (e.g. nicotine patches for smokers) or a combination of both are utilised to help affected women.

The social history is also important when planning care as women with financial issues will not be able to afford a costly therapy and those with limited home supports or physical disability may need rehabilitation post-operatively.

2.3 Examination

Examination consists of general and gynaecological components.

General examination starting with vital signs, is focussed on detecting haemo dynamic stability, thyroid dysfunction, anaemia and abdominal palpation for masses. Gynaecological examination involves inspection of the external genitalia, speculum examination of the vagina and cervix and bimanual pelvic examination.

Start your examination with three steps (ICE):

1. *Introduction*: Introduce yourself by name and position
2. *Consent*: Obtain consent to examine the woman and chaperone, if appropriate
3. *Explanation*: Explain what you are going to do as part of your examination

General examination

The general inspection begins when the woman enters the consultation room. There are four components summarised in the acronym ABCD:

1. *Appearance*: Observe the woman for the following signs:
   - Pallor indicating anaemia
   - Dysmorphic features indicating an underlying chromosomal condition
   - Neck goitre indicating hyper- or hypothyroidism
   - Discomfort or pain
2. *Body habitus*: Notice if the woman is of normal body mass index (BMI) [weight (kg)/height (m^2)]. Increased BMI is

linked to polycystic ovarian syndrome, endometrial hyperplasia/cancer and surgical morbidity. On the other hand, below average BMI is associated with amenorrhoea.

3. *Cognition*: Is the woman oriented or, as a result of severe mental or physical illness, disoriented to time, place and person?

4. *Devices/Drugs*: Does the woman have any medications with her? Does she use any treatment devices or mobilisation aids?

Vital signs

The vital signs include blood pressure, heart rate, respiratory rate, oxygen saturation and temperature.

Abdomen

Examine for a palpable fundus by placing your fully extended hand on the abdomen and use the palm and palmar surface of the fingers to identify the location, size and consistency of the fundus. A normal uterus is not palpable abdominally; however, if enlarged by a fibroid, for example, it may be palpable at a level that is even above the umbilicus.

Good practice point

A complete gynaecological examination involves the vagina and maintaining the woman's dignity is important. This can be achieved by clearly explaining what you plan to do and why, as well as offering for a chaperone to be present during the examination.

Always start your examination with less sensitive parts of the body (e.g. general and abdominal examination) as this helps patient comfort.

When examining the vulva and vagina, other body parts should always remain covered, curtains closed and doors secured to prevent inadvertent intrusion to help put the woman at ease. Similarly, an examination couch that points away from the door increases reassurance. She should be allowed the opportunity to halt the examination if and when she desires.

Clinical insight

Young women will compensate for large volumes of blood loss for quite some time before their vital signs become abnormal.

For example, be highly suspicious of a woman with a positive pregnancy test, acute abdomen (significant pain with rebound and guarding) and tachycardia, even if her blood pressure is normal.

This woman may have a ruptured ectopic and waiting until the blood pressure is low to intervene increases her morbidity, risk of mortality and laparotomy over laparoscopy.

Clinical insight

Always observe the woman's face for any grimacing when performing a potentially painful examination such as abdominal or bimanual palpation. This is not only important to ensure the woman's comfort, but also to accurately identify source and location of pain.

Next, note any surgical scars and ensure all have been accounted for in the clinical history. Look for organomegaly or masses, then examine the uterine wall and borders. Irregularities in the wall may also be caused by fibroids. If suspicious of intra-abdominal or intra-uterine pathology, palpate the abdomen to establish if there is a region of tenderness with rebound (pain upon removal of pressure) or guarding (involuntary contraction of the abdominal wall to touch) – these indicate peritoneal irritation from the presence of blood or pus.

Pelvis

As the pelvic organs, including the cervix (the opening of the uterus), are internal, visual inspection requires examination with a retraction device called a speculum. There are a number of different types of speculums for different purposes (**Figure 2.1**). Speculums are essential to observe the appearance of the cervix, perform a cervical screening test and to take high vaginal and endocervical swabs.

The pelvic organs (uterus, tubes and ovaries) are situated deep within the pelvis. This means that palpating normal pelvic organs is not possible with an abdominal examination only. Furthermore, normal pelvic organs are mobile and adequate palpation is also not possible with a digital vaginal examination alone. Therefore, in order to adequately assess the pelvic organs, a bimanual vaginal examination is required as this fixes the organ between your hands.

When both a speculum and bimanual examination are required, perform the speculum examination first so as not to disrupt the vaginal or cervical environment in case of the need to sample cervical cells or vaginal discharge.

Speculum examination

The examination is performed with either clean (most examinations) or aseptic (where sterility is required – rare in

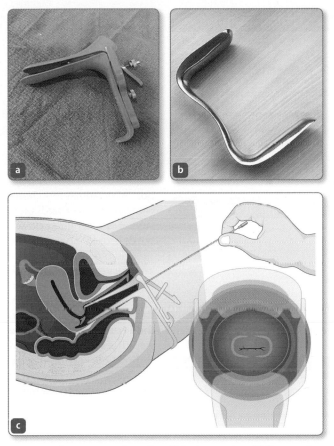

Figure 2.1 Common types of speculum. (a) Bivalve speculum; (b) Sims speculum and (c) Using a bivalve speculum.

gynaecology outside of an operating theatre) technique and by using an appropriately sized bivalve speculum (**Figure 2.1a**). A Graves speculum is wider and the edges are curved outwards. This is used in multiparous women, whereas a straighter, narrower, Pederson speculum is used in women who have not had a vaginal birth. Verbal consent is obtained and a chaperone is

Clinical insight

Ensure that the pillow or rolled up towel is placed under the woman's bottom, not under the small of her back. Placing the pillow under the bottom helps to align the vaginal canal and tilt the pelvis forwards, making visualisation of the cervix easier. If placed under the small of the back, the pelvis is tilted further backwards, making visualisation of the cervix difficult.

Clinical insight

In the past, examiners may have asked women to place their closed fists under their bottom to facilitate pelvic elevation. This is no longer recommended as this position is 'submissive' and lacks dignity. In addition, many women are unable to reach the correct position on their bottom to achieve adequate elevation.

Clinical insight

Cervical motion tenderness, formerly known as 'cervical excitation,' is positive when the patient reacts with extreme pain, withdrawing rapidly from the examiner after gentle cervical manipulation. This is indicative of significant pelvic inflammation or irritation, which may be seen with tubo-ovarian abscess or haemoperitoneum due to, for example, a ruptured ectopic pregnancy. It is analogous to rebound and guarding and occurs because the broad ligament, composed of folded pelvic peritoneum, is placed on tension by moving the cervix.

offered. The woman is asked to lie in a supine position with her bottom elevated off the examination table. Such elevation can be achieved with either a pillow or rolled up towel.

Water-based lubricant is applied to both valves of the speculum with a gloved finger. The labia are parted and the speculum is rested on the posterior vaginal fourchette with gentle downwards pressure. It is then tilted downwards on a 45° angle and the speculum gently introduced into the vagina to the length of the speculum. It is then slowly opened under vision; the cervix identified and then moved into complete view. The speculum is locked in position with a locking mechanism (generally either a valve or screw on the base), cervix inspected and any cervical sampling or swabs are taken. The speculum is then gently removed after the locking mechanism is released.

Bimanual vaginal examination

A bimanual examination is performed with the index finger and middle finger of the gloved dominant hand placed gently into the vagina into the posterior fornix and under the cervix. The non-dominant hand is placed flat on the anterior abdomen and the pelvic organs are balloted between the two. The internal fingers are rotated into each adnexa (left and right), while the external (abdominal) hand moves to push the pelvic organs onto the internal (vaginal) hand. Cervical motion tenderness is elicited by gently touching the cervix with side-to-side pressure.

In this way, the mobility, size, regularity and position of the pelvic organs can be assessed in a manner, which cannot always be achieved with other methods such as ultrasound.

2.4 Investigations

In gynaecology, there are a number of investigations that can be useful in assisting with correct diagnosis. These are selected based on the clinical presentation and the differential diagnoses that need to be included or excluded.

Haematological (blood) tests
Full blood evaluation and iron studies
A full blood evaluation (FBE) is essential to identify anaemia, which may be associated with menorrhagia. It can also identify leucocytosis, which may indicate pelvic infection or sepsis. Iron studies are useful in the evaluation of anaemia to assess for iron deficiency, which may result from menorrhagia.

C-reactive protein
C-reactive protein (CRP) is a useful marker of infection. While it is non-specific, a very high CRP (e.g. over 100) can indicate significant intra-pelvic infection and warrant further assessment.

Sex steroids (luteinising hormone, follicle-stimulating hormone, oestradiol, progesterone, and 17-hydroxy-progesterone)
These steroids are used to assess infertility and oligomenorrhoea. Follicle-stimulating hormone (FSH) can be used to identify premature ovarian failure and luteinising hormone (LH) and 17-hydroxyprogesterone can be used to assess

hyper-androgenism. Oestradiol and progesterone can act as indicators of cycle phase and ovulation, but FSH and LH also change through the cycle (e.g. both peak at ovulation).

For this reason, these tests are usually performed early in the follicular phase (around cycle day 3) where a standardised range exists as this makes interpretation easier.

Tumour markers (cancer antigen-125, inhibin and alpha-fetoprotein)

Gynaecological tumour markers can be used to assess some gynaecological cancers. Sometimes, other tumour markers [e.g. carcinoembryonic antigen (CEA) and cancer antigen 19-9 (CA 19-9)] are also ordered to assess for the possibility of a non-gynaecological primary malignancy or metastasis. Cancer antigen-125 (CA-125) is a non-specific tumour marker, which can be raised in epithelial ovarian cancers. Inhibin is raised in granulosa cell ovarian cancers and alpha-fetoprotein (AFP) is raised in immature teratomas. CA 19-9 is raised in upper gastrointestinal malignancy but can also be raised with ovarian dermoids and mucinous borderline tumours.

Beta-human chorionic gonadotropin

Serum quantitative beta-human chorionic gonadotropin (β-hCG) is an essential tool in assessing pregnancy status. It can also be used to track an ectopic pregnancy and its response to medical treatment (see Chapter 6). Choriocarcinomas (ovarian and persistent gestational trophoblast) also release β-hCG and this is a useful marker to assess treatment response.

> ### Good practice point
>
> Cancer antigen-125 is non-specific and can also be raised in several benign conditions including endometriosis. A raised CA-125 by itself does not necessarily indicate cancer. It is not recommended to perform tumour markers in the presence of normal imaging for this reason or 'blindly' as a screening test.

Imaging tests

Imaging is an essential part of the gynaecological assessment. Transvaginal ultrasound is the single most useful imaging modality in gynaecology. For more complicated situations, CT scanning and MRI may be required.

Transvaginal ultrasound

Because of the proximity of the pelvic organs to the vagina, a transvaginal ultrasound is the most effective approach to imaging the uterus, tubes and ovaries. This is because a close probe can use a high frequency which given superior spatial resolution.

In children, a transvaginal ultrasound is not appropriate. In these circumstances, a transabdominal or translabial ultrasound may suffice.

Ultrasound can image in real-time and assess size of pelvic organs, tenderness, pelvic fluid, vascularity and the nature of many pathologies including fibroids, polyps and ovarian cysts.

CT of the abdomen/pelvis

Usually reserved for excluding non-gynaecological causes of abdominal pain, a CT of the abdomen/pelvis may incidentally find a pelvic pathology such as an ovarian mass. In these circumstances, it is always worthwhile obtaining a dedicated pelvic transvaginal ultrasound to further characterise any pelvic lesions.

A CT is also sometimes used in the assessment of gynaeco-logical cancers and metastasis as a staging test (to determine how far spread the cancer is in the body).

MRI of the pelvis

Usually, MRI is reserved for imaging assessment of cervical cancer and malignant spread, as it can identify parametrial and paravesical and rectal pathology well and this is where cervical cancer spreads. Occasionally, MRI is also used in the assessment of uterine sarcoma or advanced endometriosis. MR-guided ultrasound can also be used to treat fibroids.

Procedural investigations

In order to provide a complete assessment, procedural diag-nostic tests sometimes need to be employed. These have the benefit of direct visualisation of pathology as well as providing tissue samples for histological analysis.

Office endometrial sampling

In most women, an endometrial sample can be obtained in the office using an aspiration catheter (e.g. Pipelle) (**Figure 2.2**). This provides a core of endometrial tissue, which can be sent for histological analysis. This is done without direct vision of the endometrial cavity, but is limited as it only samples a small proportion of the endometrium. It is not suitable where focal pathology such as a polyp is suspected or where the cervix is very narrow.

Diagnostic hysteroscopy

While ultrasound and variations of ultrasound (including saline hysterography) are effective at identifying intrauterine lesions (e.g. polyps and fibroids), they may not give an accurate description of uterine synechiae (scarring) or uterine anomalies such as septae. In addition, they cannot delineate cavity involvement in all cases.

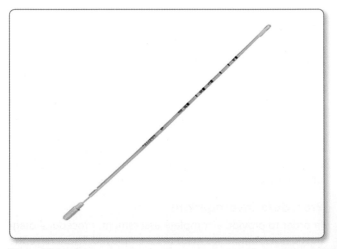

Figure 2.2 Pipelle.

This is where diagnostic hysteroscopy performs well as it permits direct visualisation. Additionally, hysteroscopy allows simultaneous treatment. This makes it preferred over separate specialised ultrasound tests such as saline infusion, if such pathology (e.g. polyps) is suspected.

Diagnostic laparoscopy

Intra-abdominal pathology, such as endometriosis, may be small in size or flat and may not be visualised accurately on imaging. The gold standard assessment for endometriosis is laparoscopy. While this is an operative intervention, the benefits of diagnostic laparoscopy in someone with pelvic pain cannot be under-estimated as long as it is followed on by appropriate treatment.

Puberty and congenital disorders

3.1 Introduction

Puberty is a time of physiological and psychological change. It also coincides with the psychosocial transition from childhood to adult roles, desires and experiences, and for this reason is one of the most challenging life phases we navigate.

This chapter outlines normal pubertal development, the most common disorders of puberty and developmental abnormalities of the female reproductive tract.

3.2 Clinical scenario

Presentation

Chloe, a 16-year-old girl, attends with her mother for your advice. She has not started menstruating. Her mother is concerned as her own periods started at the age of 13 years.

In response to your questioning, Chloe reports that she is taller than her peers, has had breast development for the last 4 years, minimal pubic hair, and has not noticed cyclic abdominal pain or an abdominal mass. She is medically healthy and her body mass index (BMI) is 19 kg/m^2. She does not exercise excessively and her childhood development and milestones are normal. She has usual levels of stress associated with school.

There is no other family history of significance. Chloe has a younger sister, 10 years, who is well and not yet pubertal. An aunt adopted two children due to infertility, but the family do not know further details. Physical examination and external genital inspection are normal.

Diagnostic approach

Delayed menarche has a wide differential, the most common being normal, but slower than average, progress. This is termed 'constitutional'. Pathological causes include:

- Central hypothalamic delay due to stress, exercise, systemic disease or low BMI

- Premature gonadal failure due to genetic, structural, infective or iatrogenic causes, and
- Absent or abnormal uterine development

Absence of menses 2 years after breast development and lack of menses at the age of 16 years are abnormal and warrant further investigation.

Further investigations

Minimum key information required to differentiate between the possible causes above is gonadotropin [luteinising hormone (LH) and follicle-stimulating hormone (FSH)] levels (elevated, normal or low), karyotype (XX or abnormal) and whether or not a uterus and ovaries are present.

Chloe's hormonal profile shows physiological FSH and LH. Pelvic ultrasound reveals an absent uterus and gonads that are located in the inguinal canal bilaterally. Karyotype is 46,XY. Androgens are completed and are in the physiological male range.

A diagnosis of complete androgen insensitivity syndrome (CAIS) is made.

Management

Chloe and her mother are informed of the diagnosis sensitively with particular emphasis that this does not mean male gender, as women with CAIS are, apart from absent uterus, phenotypically and psychosocially female.

The short- and long-term issues with this syndrome are discussed, including gonadectomy for malignancy risk and psychological implications. Fertility and family planning issues are introduced with the understanding that these will become more important in later years. Chloe's younger sister is offered her own assessment and karyotype, as the condition is heritable in an X-linked recessive manner and Chloe's mother is, therefore, a carrier.

Importantly, opportunity for further discussion is offered as well as referral to specialty care and support groups.

While CAIS is rare, the approach to disorders of puberty allows logical identification of this condition.

3.3 Physiology of normal puberty

Normal puberty is a complex biological and psychological event. Puberty has three key components: (1) adrenarche (secretion of adrenal androgens and sexual hair growth), (2) thelarche (breast growth), and (3) menarche (menstruation).

Adrenarche occurs due to adrenal axis maturation with production of androgen hormones, whereas thelarche and menarche both occur due to oestrogen released by the ovaries as a result of maturation of the hypothalamic-pituitary axis (**Figure 3.1**).

Normal pubertal sequence

The onset of thelarche typically precedes adrenarche, which is then followed by menarche 1–2 years later. Typical ages for adrenarche and thelarche are 9–12 years and menarche are 11–14 years; however, the normal range is wide (**Figure 3.2**).

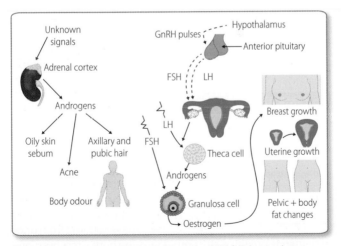

Figure 3.1 Adrenarche and thelarche/menarche. (FSH, follicle-stimulating hormone; GnRH, gonadotropin-releasing hormone; LH, luteinising hormone)

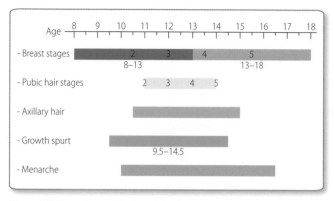

Figure 3.2 Normal range of pubertal development.

Guiding principle

Adrenarche before the age of 8 years and thelarche/menarche before the age of 9 years are considered abnormal (premature). A lack of any pubertal development by the age of 14 years, or menstruation 2 years after development of breasts or by the age of 16 years is considered delayed puberty.

Clinical insight

In females, circulating androgen levels are much lower than male levels and by adulthood, the ovaries and adrenal glands equally release androgens. This is unlike in males, where gonadal androgen production, predominantly testosterone, is much higher. Female adolescents tend to have less severe acne for this reason.

Adrenarche

The biological trigger for adrenarche has not been established; however, adrenal androgen production, particularly of dehydroepiandrosterone sulphate (DHEAS), increases from the age of 10 years. This is progressively supplemented by the other main source of endogenous androgens, which are produced in the ovaries.

Circulating androgens cause several physical changes as outlined in **Table 3.1**.

Adrenarche occurs earlier in children who are obese or who have suffered from prior intrauterine growth restriction suggesting both stress hormone and weight-related triggers are important.

Area	Effect
Skin	Sebum production (androgen receptor-bearing skin in, particular, the face, chest and interscapular region) and acne
Head hair	Oily (due to sebum production)
Axillae	• Apocrine secretion from androgen receptor-bearing glands – body odour as axillary bacteria break these compounds into malodorous metabolites • Hair growth (androgen receptor-bearing hair follicles)
Genitalia	• Darkening • Hair growth, initially over labia and spreading gradually over mons

Table 3.1 Effects of androgens

Thelarche and menarche

Hypothalamic-pituitary-ovarian axis activation starts in the pituitary gland with development of gonadotropin-releasing hormone (GnRH) pulses, initially nocturnal, causing a rise in FSH and LH and a small rise in serum oestrogen.

Clinical insight

Adrenarche and thelarche/menarche have different controls. In disordered puberty, these may be activated separately. For this reason, a pubertal history should establish the timeline of what has developed and when.

Oestrogen causes the breasts to begin developing (breast bud), the uterus to grow and the endometrium to thicken. Eventually, GnRH pulses occur throughout the day and night and oestrogen concentrations rise further. At this point, endometrial shedding and menarche occur (**Figure 3.3**).

In parallel with these gonadal axis changes, growth hormone secretion rises. This causes a period of rapid skeletal growth culminating in the achievement of final adult height. Growth then stops because the long bone epiphyses (the part of the bone where new bone can be formed to lengthen it) fuse under the influence of adult oestrogen concentrations.

Regular menstrual cycles develop over time as the hypothalamic-pituitary-ovarian axis matures. The menstrual cycle then has a first half with follicular recruitment and oestrogen

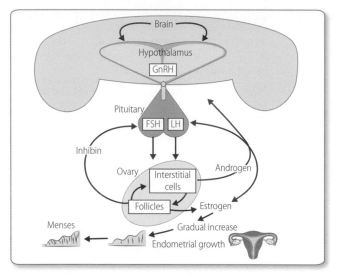

Figure 3.3 HPO activation/menarche. (FSH,: follicle-stimulating hormone; GnRH, gonadotropin-releasing hormone; HPO, hypothalamic-pituitary-ovarian; LH, luteinising hormone)

Clinical insight

The first 12 menstrual cycles are frequently anovulatory, as control of the gonadal axis is immature. Menses are often irregular and are less painful than in ovulatory cycles, as uterine prostaglandin production requires the effect of progesterone, which will only be found if ovulation takes place.

For this reason, primary dysmenorrhoea, painful menses due to prostaglandin production develops after menarche usually by around 12–24 months and is best treated by prostaglandin inhibition using anti-inflammatory medications and/or suppressing ovulation with the oral contraceptive pill.

production stimulated by FSH. In the mid-cycle, high oestrogen results in a LH 'surge' which stimulates ovulation. After ovulation, progesterone production from the corpus luteum marks the second half of the menstrual cycle.

The length of the first half of the cycle is variable as the time taken to recruit a lead follicle and reach adequate oestrogen levels to trigger ovulation varies. However, the length of the second half of the cycle is fairly constant at 12–14 days, as this is the lifespan of the corpus luteum, which produces the post-ovulatory progesterone. In the absence of pregnancy, the withdrawal of this progesterone results in menstruation, oestrogen also falls and the cycle begins anew.

The development of breasts follows five stages (the 'Tanner' stages) (**Figure 3.4**). Together with the development of sexual hair, puberty can be objectively 'staged' and described in terms of Tanner stage for breasts and hair. Stage 1 refers to pre-pubertal appearance (no breast development or sexual hair) and stage 5 refers to adult female appearance. Stages 2, 3 and 4 are differentiated by development of breast bud,

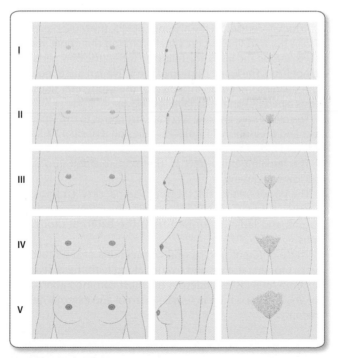

Figure 3.4 Tanner staging.

early sexual hair and areolar projection above the mature breast, respectively.

3.4 Physiology of normal female genital development

In normal early embryonic development, there are two primitive internal genital systems – the Müllerian and Wolffian ducts. The Müllerian duct forms female internal genitalia and the Wolffian duct forms male internal genitalia and the vas deferens. Müllerian development and fusion are prevented in male fetuses by the production of Müllerian inhibiting substance (MIS) in the fetal testis and fetal testosterone promotes development of internal male genitals from the Wolffian ducts (**Figure 3.5**).

In female fetuses, in the absence of MIS, the Müllerian ducts fuse in the mid-line, progressively forming the upper vagina, cervix, uterus and lastly, the fallopian tubes (the only parts that do not fuse). The lower portion of the Müllerian ducts, now the upper vagina, meets an infolding of the urogenital sinus and forms a patent vaginal canal (**Figure 3.6**).

The ovaries are entirely separate structures to the Müllerian duct and their normal formation relies on a normal XX karyotype and blood supply.

The female genital tract is, therefore, divided into upper and lower segments.

The upper genital tract (upper vagina, cervix, uterus and fallopian tubes) is of Müllerian origin. The lower genital tract (vagina and labia) is formed from the external urogenital sinus.

These different origins and connections of the Müllerian ducts, urogenital sinus and ovaries along with the absence of MIS from fetal testes underpin the most common abnormalities you will encounter in female internal and external genital anatomy.

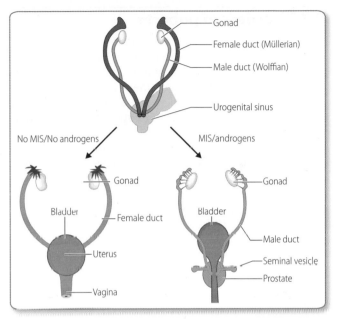

Figure 3.5 Müllerian and Wolffian ducts. (MIS, Müllerian inhibiting substance)

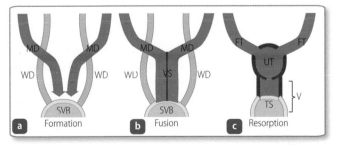

Figure 3.6 Formation of uterus and vagina. [FT, fallopian tube; MD, Müllerian duct; SVB, sinovaginal bulb (developing vagina); TS, transverse septum; UT, uterus; V, vagina; VS, vertical septum; WD, Wolffian duct]

3.5 Disorders of puberty

The three major pubertal disorders are too early (premature), too late (delayed) or in the wrong sequence (and usually too early). Most of the causes are benign and associated with good prognosis with treatment. Treatment avoids psychosocial consequences and short final stature as the epiphyses close in response to early exposure to sex steroids (oestrogen and androgens).

Rarely, pubertal development may go awry in other manners including male pattern development, 'virilisation' (growth of clitoris, beard hair and voice deepening normally associated with male puberty). This is very rare and always pathological.

> **Clinical insight**
>
> Premature puberty occurs much more commonly in girls than boys at a ratio of 5:1.

This section will focus on premature pubertal and delayed pubertal conditions, their diagnosis and management.

Premature puberty
Definition

Premature puberty is defined as pubertal development before the age of 8 years in girls. This can present as isolated thelarche, adrenarche or complete pubertal sequence.

Differential diagnosis

Premature puberty can either be central, meaning the puberty is due to early secretion of FSH/LH from the brain or peripheral, meaning the puberty is due to peripheral production of oestrogen or androgen when it should not be occurring as the brain has not sent the appropriate signal (FSH/LH). Central puberty is the most common form and also most commonly idiopathic (75% of cases).

Peripheral premature puberty is always pathological. The groups are compared in **Table 3.2**.

History

History taking aims to establish the sequence, timeline and rate of progress of pubertal development. Enquire about which

Type	Features	Causes	Findings
Central precocious puberty	• 'Gonadotropin dependent' caused by GnRH and FSH/LH • Premature physiological pubertal levels of FSH/LH and oestrogen • No virilising signs are present • Premature breast development • Premature menstruation • Period of skeletal growth followed by permanent short stature (epiphyseal closure) • Premature acne, body odour and sexual hair if accompanied by adrenarche	• Idiopathic (75%) • Brain tumour, e.g. hamartoma • Brain radiotherapy • Central nervous system (CNS) malformation • May be associated with IUGR, psychosocial stress and obesity	• FSH* and LH in adult female range • Oestradiol in adult female range • DHEAS in adult female range, if adrenarche exists • Advanced bone age on wrist X-ray • ±Abnormal CNS imaging (hamartoma, tumour, hydrocephalus and others) • Common to all
Peripheral precocious puberty	• 'Gonadotropin independent,' not a consequence of GnRH/FSH/LH – either oestrogen producing or androgen producing • Premature pubertal levels of oestrogen or androgens but not FSH/LH • Virilising signs, if androgen producing cause • Premature breast development • Premature menstruation • Period of skeletal growth followed by permanent short stature (epiphyseal closure) • Premature acne and body odour and sexual hair, if androgen producing cause	• Pathological • Oestrogen-secreting ovarian tumour (benign, germ cell and others) • Exogenous oestrogen consumption • Adrenal tumour – usually with virilising signs • CAH – usually with virilising signs • McCune–Albright syndrome – associated with café-au-lait spots • Hypothyroidism (severe – usually with other signs and symptoms)	• FSH and LH are very low • ↑ Oestradiol • ↑ Testosterone • ↑ DHEAS (CAH) • ↑ 17-OHP (CAH) • Advanced bone age on wrist X-ray • Elevated TSH (hypothyroidism) • Ovarian or adrenal tumour

(DHEAS, dehydroepiandrosterone sulphate; FSH, follicle-stimulating hormone GnRH, gonadotropin-releasing hormone; IUGR, intrauterine growth restriction; LH, luteinising hormone; 17-OHP, 17-hydroxyprogesterone; TSH, thyroid-stimulating hormone; CNS, central nervous system; CAH, congenital adrenal hyperplasia)
*FSH levels alone are not discriminatory, as they can vary considerably and overlap between prepubertal and pubertal results. LH is reliable.

Table 3.2 Premature puberty

symptom was noted first (thelarche, breast bud vs. adrenarche, odour and hair vs. menarche and vaginal bleeding), progression of puberty, rate and linear skeletal growth.

Parental pubertal age is useful, as it is a heritable trait and many 'idiopathic' premature puberties follow a familial course.

Also ask about virilizing symptoms (male pattern development), as these suggest a peripheral pathological cause. Enquire regarding access to sex steroid medication (commonly oral contraceptives or hormone replacement), neurological symptoms and symptoms of hypothyroidism as well as presence of café-au-lait spots (McCune–Albright syndrome) to exclude other major differentials in central and peripheral precocious puberty.

Examination

Examination aims to identify the potential cause and stage of puberty. Key examination steps and findings are shown in **Table 3.3**.

Take note of general appearance (acne, seborrhoea and odour) and measure height, weight and BMI. Perform a neurological examination, if a central nervous system (CNS) tumour is suspected on history. Examine the neck for a goitre (hypothyroidism).

Perform Tanner staging of the breasts and external genitalia, as this will enable you to be systematic in your description for later comparison.

Examine the abdomen for masses (tumours).

The physical findings should be summarised as either premature adrenarche, thelarche, menarche or puberty (all components).

Investigations

Investigations aim to determine if the puberty is due to central gonadotropin release or peripheral pathology. Therefore, perform serum FSH/LH and oestradiol as baseline (**Table 3.4**).

Complete adrenal (DHEAS) and gonadal (testosterone) androgens in those with signs of androgen exposure or

	Findings	Significance
Appearance	Oily hair/skin	Adrenarche
Height, weight and BMI	• Taller than peers • Obesity	• Accelerated skeletal growth – risk of epiphyseal closure • Common association of 'idiopathic'
Skin	• Acne • Beard area hair • Café-au-lait spots	• Adrenarche or peripheral testosterone production • Virilisation (CAH and tumours) • McCune–Albright syndrome
Neck	Goitre	Hypothyroidism
Chest	Breast development	Oestrogen exposure
Abdomen	Mass 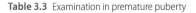	Ovarian cyst
Genitalia	• Menses • Pubic hair • Clitoromegaly	• Oestrogen exposure • Adrenarche or peripheral testosterone exposure • Virilisation (CAH and tumours)

(BMI, body mass index; CAH, congenital adrenal hyperplasia)

Table 3.3 Examination in premature puberty

virilisation together with 17-hydroxyprogesterone, as this will detect adrenarche, androgen-producing tumours and congenital adrenal hyperplasia.

> **Clinical insight**
>
> Isolated premature thelarche or adrenarche can be safely observed, as they will not cause stunted final height.

A wrist X-ray will establish bone age by the degree of ossification in the carpal bones and radius/ulna, as they ossify in a characteristic sequence and age.

Children with neurological signs or symptoms should also have CNS imaging by MRI.

Management

The key principles are to:
• Delay premature sexual development

Conditions	FSH/LH	Oestradiol	Progesterone	Testosterone	Other androgens (DHEAS and 17-OHP)
Central premature puberty	Post-pubertal range	Post-pubertal range	Post-pubertal range	Normal female range	Normal female range
Peripheral premature puberty	Pre-pubertal range (low)	↑If oestrogen secreting cause		↑If testosterone secreting cause	↑If secreting cause, e.g. CAH and tumours
Pseudo-puberty (medication consumption)	Low	Low	Low	Low	Low

(CAH, congenital adrenal hyperplasia; DHEAS, dehydroepiandrosterone sulphate; FSH, follicle-stimulating hormone; LH, luteinising hormone; 17-OHP, 17-hydroxyprogesterone)

Table 3.4 Gonadal axis patterns in abnormal puberty

- Prevent early epiphyseal closure
- Treat the cause of pathological central and peripheral puberty

Idiopathic central precocious puberty is treated by using gonadotropin downregulating medications to suppress early FSH/LH release, until an appropriate age is reached for puberty to occur, at which time these medications are ceased.

Delayed puberty

Definition

Pubertal delay can be primary (no pubertal development) or secondary/arrest (cessation of puberty after starting). Primary pubertal delay is investigated at the age of 14 years and secondary pubertal delay with absence of menses by the age of 16 years or 2 years from breast development should also be investigated.

Differential diagnosis

The two main groups of delay are lack of FSH/LH signals from the brain (hypogonadotropic) and inability for the body to respond to FSH/LH signals (hypergonadotropic).

Eugonadotropic delay occurs where FSH and LH concentrations are normal, is always secondary and affects menses (**Table 3.5**).

History and examination

History and examination in a girl with pubertal delay should focus on identifying dysmorphism (hypergonadotropic causes include genetic syndromes), the presence of partial pubertal development (perform Tanner staging) and a confirmation of parental age of puberty (to identify constitutional delay).

Also enquire regarding menopausal symptoms in cases of partial pubertal sequence (breasts without menses), as this strongly suggests hypergonadotropic ovarian failure such as in Turner syndrome.

Gonads can be palpated in the inguinal canal in CAIS (undescended testes). An imperforate hymen can be seen as a genital bulge with blue-black blood above with an enlarged uterus is palpated abdominally.

	Hypogonadotropic	Hypergonadotropic	Eugonadotropic
Causes	• Constitutional • Stress, dieting and excessive exercise	• Genetic syndromes – Turner syndrome (45, XO), other including Swyer syndrome (46, XY) • Ovarian agenesis/dysgenesis • Ovarian injury – radiation, chemotherapy, surgery, autoimmune and idiopathic premature failure	• Genetic syndromes – CAIS (46 XY) • Developmental syndromes – MA – 46, XX • Developmental syndromes – IH
FSH/LH	↓	←	Normal
Oestradiol	↓	→	Normal
Ovaries	Normal	Abnormal	Testes in CAIS Present in MA + IH
Uterus	Present	Present	Absent – CAIS and MA Present – IH
Breasts	Absent	Absent	Present

(FSH, follicle-stimulating hormone; LH, luteinising hormone; MA, Müllerian agenesis; CAIS, complete androgen insensitivity syndrome; IH, imperforate hymen)

Table 3.5 Types of abnormal pubertal delay

Hypogonadotropic delay Hypogonadotropic delay is the most common cause. Most cases are constitutional, i.e. development will occur normally albeit later than average. This is a familial trait.

Other cases are due to having a low BMI, which is inadequate to promote normal development. This is usually due to behavioural factors such as eating disorders or excessive exercise and is reversible.

Girls with hypogonadotropic delay, therefore, have a good prognosis and she can be reassured regarding ultimate development and future fertility.

Eugonadotropic delay Eugonadotropic (normal FSH and LH levels) delay always occurs as a secondary finding with partial pubertal development (breasts present and absent menses).

This is found with CAIS, Müllerian (uterine) agenesis and Imperforate hymen, as either the uterus is absent or menses obstructed and no periods occur.

Complete androgen insensitivity syndrome In CAIS, an androgen receptor gene mutation renders it non-functional. This does not affect females (XX), but a genetic male fetus (XY) cannot respond to testosterone and develops a female phenotype. The uterus is absent, as development is inhibited by the presence of MIS from the fetal testes. In adolescence, partial female puberty occurs as testicular testosterone is metabolized to oestrogen in peripheral tissues. There is little, if any, sexual hair as the hair-bearing skin is unable to respond to androgens.

Individuals with CAIS frequently present with normal breast development, scanty genital hair and primary amenorrhoea.

Müllerian agenesis In Müllerian agenesis, the uterus in a genetic female fails to develop early in embryonic life for unknown reasons; however, all else is normal including the ovaries. Puberty is, therefore, normal apart from primary amenorrhoea.

Imperforate hymen In imperforate hymen, failure of normal canalisation (the fetal breakdown of the membrane between the developing vagina and upper Müllerian-derived genital

Clinical insight

Menopausal symptoms (hot flushes and night sweats) are only experienced by those who have had exposure to oestrogen before it is lost. Therefore, girls with primary failure of puberty will not experience these symptoms, despite very low oestrogen levels, but girls with gonadal failure after starting puberty will experience these symptoms.

tract) results in obstructed menses. This causes cyclical pain, uterine enlargement with trapped blood and development of a palpable abdominal mass due to the distended uterus. Endometriosis can also occur from retrograde menses through patent fallopian tubes.

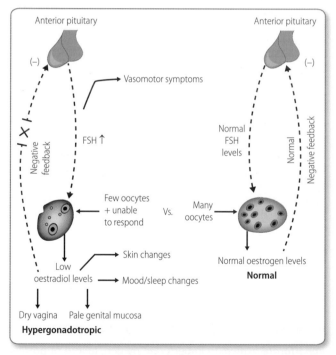

Figure 3.7 Hypergonadotropic hypogonadism.

Hypergonadotropic delay Hypergonadotropic hypogonadism reflects a permanent inability of the ovaries to respond to FSH/LH. Therefore, they do not produce oestrogen (**Figure 3.7**).

This usually happens before pubertal development, but can occur after some development as occurred. In Turner syndrome, e.g. up to 30% will have partial pubertal development before the abnormal ovary fails and oestrogen levels fall.

Investigations

Perform FSH/LH and oestradiol to differentiate hypergonadotropic from hypogonadotropic causes because management differs significantly between the two groups.

Hypergonadotropic women should also have a karyotype and pelvic ultrasound (to assess for the presence and development of gonads). In addition, a bone age X-ray is used to confirm constitutional delay (bone age also delayed).

Management

The approach to management is outlined in **Table 3.6**.

3.6 Congenital abnormalities of the female genital tract

Anomalies of internal genital midline fusion, canalisation of the upper and lower vaginal connection as well as of the gonads occur and are grouped into those with a chromosomal cause and those with a structural cause (below).

Chromosomal causes

Genetic problems can cause several malformations of the genital tract and ovaries. The most common examples include Turner syndrome (45,XO), Swyer syndrome (46,XY female) and CAIS.

Complete androgen insensitivity syndrome has been introduced above and all three conditions are summarised in **Table 3.7**.

Group	Causes	Management
Hypogonado-tropic	Constitutional	Reassure normal outcomes
	Stress, dieting and excessive exercise	• Encourage normal eating and exercise levels – natural puberty will result • If not possible – low-dose slowly titrated oestrogen until bleeding occurs then add cyclic progesterone/switch to oral contraceptive pill for hormone replacement (prevents osteoporosis and induces puberty) • Normal fertility, if provoking factor is corrected
Hypergonado-tropic	Turner syndrome (45,XO)	• Induce puberty as above • Screen for associated cardiac and renal malformations (echocardiogram and ultrasound) and thyroid disease • Family building through adoption or donor oocyte in vitro fertilization (IVF) and use of gestational surrogate if cardiac disease (risk of death increased in pregnancy) • Long-term, treat as for premature menopause with bone mineral density screening, dyslipidemia and diabetes screening
	Swyer syndrome (46,XY)	• Induce puberty as above • Gonadectomy at diagnosis (30% risk of malignancy) • Family building through adoption or donor oocyte IVF
	• Ovarian agenesis/dysgenesis • Ovarian injury – radiation, chemotherapy, surgery, autoimmune and idiopathic premature failure	• Induce puberty as above • Family building through adoption or donor oocyte IVF

Table 3.6 Management of delayed puberty. *Continues opposite.*

Group	Causes	Management
Eugonado-tropic	Genetic syndromes – complete androgen insensitivity syndrome (CAIS) (46XY)	• Allow testes to facilitate spontaneous breast development (testosterone is converted to oestrogen in the body – natural breast development) • Gonadectomy at the age of 20–25 years (malignancy risk is less than Swyer syndrome) • Family building through adoption or gestational surrogacy with donor oocyte
	Developmental syndromes – Müllerian (uterine) agenesis (MA) – 46XX	• Puberty will occur normally with primary amenorrhoea (no uterus and normal ovaries) • Family building through adoption, gestational surrogacy with own oocyte or uterine transplant
Other points	• Psychological support • Dedicated clinic	• High rates of psychosocial issues and need for support • Where possible, it facilitates optimal management

Table 3.6 *Continued*

Syndrome	Cause	Pathology	Findings
Turner syndrome	Loss of an X chromosome in embryonic formation, karyotype 45,XO	• Abnormal gonadal development, streak ovaries which fail in infancy or early adolescence • Normal uterus and vaginal development in utero • Loss of X chromosome genes	• Absent or arrested puberty due to early ovarian failure. Residual streak gonads on imaging • Normal female internal and external genitalia • Characteristic physical traits (short stature, co-arctation of aorta, cardiac defects, horseshoe kidney, webbed neck and exaggerated carrying angle of elbow)
Swyer syndrome	Loss of sex-determining region of Y chromosome, 46,XY individual	• No Müllerian inhibiting substance • Undifferentiated gonads	• Müllerian ducts develop normal female upper and lower genital tract structures • No Wolffian structures or male genitalia, as no testosterone production. Risk of gonadoblastoma in gonads
Complete androgen insensitivity syndrome (CAIS)	Mutation of androgen receptor gene on X chromosome, XY karyotype	• Inability to respond to androgen production • Testis present, with normal androgen production • Testis present, with Müllerian inhibiting substance production	• Androgen cannot act on tissues and no fetal masculinisation possible. Female fetal phenotype and external genitalia form • Müllerian ducts regress, no uterus, cervix, fallopian tubes or upper vagina. Wolffian ducts remain

Table 3.7 Chromosomal gonadal/genital abnormalities

Structural causes

The midline fusion of the Müllerian ducts and the meeting of the Müllerian ducts with the urogenital sinus are two sites of developmental errors and malformations.

Müllerian duct fusion

Errors in Müllerian duct fusion include maldevelopment of one side (unilateral hypogenesis/agenesis) and failure of normal fusion. These are illustrated in **Figure 3.8**.

These malformations are common, often incidentally diagnosed and mostly associated with normal health and reproductive outcomes. There is an association with preterm labour and malpresentation, as the uterus is functionally smaller, but this is not an inevitable outcome and you can be reassuring in your counselling.

The only exception is a septate uterus, as the septum is relatively avascular and the poor blood supply increases the risk of miscarriage if the embryo implants in this area. To

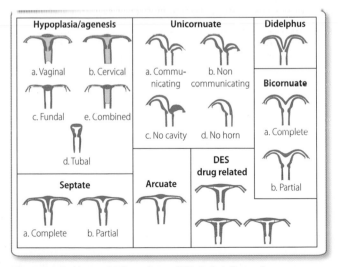

Figure 3.8 Problems in Müllerian fusion. (DES: diethylstilbestrol)

reduce this risk, resection of the septum can be performed hysteroscopically.

A septate vagina is treated by resection if it causes menstrual or sexual problems. All women with two cervixes require cervical screening from each side.

The Müllerian duct formation and renal formation are closely related. Therefore, in women with Müllerian genesis problems, it is important to arrange a renal tract ultrasound scan to ensure co-existent renal malformation that does not exist, as this may need long-term monitoring or treatment.

Urogenital sinus fusion

Another site of common developmental error is where the Müllerian duct meets the urogenital sinus. The major problems include failure of canalisation (breakdown of the epithelium separating the vagina from perineum), called imperforate hymen, and a more extensive failure of fusion, which leaves a horizontal vaginal septum.

Differentiating the two conditions is important as imperforate hymen is cured by simple surgical cruciate incision, whereas a horizontal vaginal septum requires special surgical techniques to remove the tissue to avoid stenosis.

Both conditions present with symptoms of obstructed menstruation including cyclical pelvic pain (with menstrual flow that is entrapped) and, if not identified and treated, an abdominal mass from uterine enlargement with blood. Endometriosis is more common in this population due to excessive backflow of blood through the fallopian tubes. Both conditions have excellent long-term prognosis once treated surgically.

Disorders of the menstrual cycle

4.1 Introduction

Women spend a large proportion of their adult life menstruating. This physiological event starts in adolescence, often contributing to the self-doubt and anxiety of this life stage, and finishes in the early 50s. There are very few natural breaks apart from pregnancy and breastfeeding during this time.

The number of menstrual cycles modern women have is historically unheralded. Even a few hundred years ago later menarche, high childbearing rates and reduced life expectancy meant most women had a fraction of the menstrual cycles that are now normal. Menstruation-related issues and consequences of excess menstrual events are the most common gynaecological complaints and, therefore, an understanding of the physiology and the ability to manage problems effectively is essential.

4.2 Clinical scenario

A 48-year-old gravida 3, para 2 attends for review. She reports excessively heavy menstruation for the last 5 years and complains of fatigue. There has been recent onset of decreased exercise tolerance and palpitations.

She is obese [body mass index (BMI) 40 kg/m^2] and has medicated hypertension, but is otherwise healthy and there is no other history of note. Medications include amlodipine, iron supplementation and tranexamic acid, which was recently initiated by her GP. Clinical assessment reveals an overweight woman with conjunctival pallor. The abdomen is soft with a palpable suprapubic mass. Bimanual examination confirms this to be uterine in origin.

Diagnostic approach

Menorrhagia is common in peri-menopausal women. Causes include ovulatory dysfunction, as the oocyte pool falls as well as structural pathology including adenomyosis, fibroids, polyps and endometrial hyperplasia or malignancy. The palpable uterus in this case makes structural pathology such as fibroids the most likely diagnosis although the others still require exclusion.

Investigations aim to determine the cause, severity and consequence of menorrhagia and therefore, include an assessment of haemoglobin and hematinic (substances required for production of red blood cells, iron in particular) status, uterine size and endometrial thickness. Endometrial sampling, either surgically at hysteroscopy or via outpatient Pipelle endometrial biopsy, is required in order to conclusively exclude endometrial malignancy.

Clinical insight

Menorrhagia is a common problem at both ends of the reproductive spectrum; however, the causes are different. Early post-menarchal girls frequently have anovulatory cycles as their hypothalamic-gonadal axis is immature. This results in endometrial overgrowth and irregular heavy shedding. They respond well to medical management to provide progesterone stabilisation of the endometrium. Peri-menopausal women frequently have structural pathology and, if this is confirmed, are more likely to elect for surgery to address this.

Guiding principle

Any woman over the age of 45 years with persistent heavy periods or of any age with a thickened endometrium >16 mm requires histological sampling of the endometrium to exclude endometrial hyperplasia (a pre-malignant change) and endometrial malignancy.

Further investigations

Haematological investigations reveal iron deficiency anaemia with a haemoglobin of 87 g/L and ferritin of 5 μg/L. Ultrasound confirms the presence of an enlarged fibroid uterus with distortion of the endometrial cavity. The endometrial thickness is within normal limits at 12 mm. Pipelle endometrial biopsy is benign.

Management

The woman is counselled regarding her medical and surgical options for her heavy bleeding and elects for hysterectomy. Her haemoglobin is optimised pre-operatively with intravenous iron and bleeding is controlled temporarily with oral progesterone.

She undergoes an open abdominal procedure as her uterus is too large for laparoscopic removal and does not descend enough for a vaginal approach. Her ovaries are conserved, but fallopian tubes are removed. She makes an uneventful recovery.

4.3 Menstrual cycle disturbance

A menstrual cycle starts on the first day of menses (cycle day 1) and ends on the last day before the next menses (typically day 28). Variation of a few days is normal.

As outlined in Chapter 1, the normal menstrual cycle ranges from 21 to 35 days with 3–6 days of bleeding and once regular menses are established, minimal variation between cycles of up to 2–3 days.

Cycles outside of this are defined as abnormal but a small number of otherwise healthy women will have cycles outside the above values. In the absence of pathological cause or bother, treatment is not required.

Disorders of the menstrual cycle fall into three main categories:
1. Disorders of cycle length
2. Disorders of cycle regularity
3. Disorders of bleeding heaviness

Disorders of cycle length include cycles that are too short with menstruation occurring shorter than 21 days apart (polymenorrhoea), cycles that are too long with menstruation occurring greater than 35 days apart (oligomenorrhoea) and cycles that do not occur at all (amenorrhoea).

Disorders of cycle regularity are called metrorrhagia if the bleeding is irregular, and metromenorrhagia if the bleeding is also heavy.

Disorders of bleeding heaviness include unusually light menstruation (hypomenorrhoea) and overly heavy menstruation (menorrhagia).

Of the disorders, the most frequent presentations are for menorrhagia and metromenorhagia. This is because heavy or irregular bleeding is more likely to impact quality of life and cause complications including iron deficiency anaemia. Like endometriosis and pelvic pain disorders, menorrhagia causes significant psychological, social, financial and quality of life issues and complaints should be taken seriously.

Amenorrhoea
Definitions
Amenorrhoea refers to the absence of menstrual periods and has two main types: (1) primary and (2) secondary.

Primary amenorrhoea exists when an adolescent has not had menstrual bleeding by the age of 16 years. Once menstrual cycles occur, secondary amenorrhoea is defined as 3 months without menses in a previously regularly cycling women and 6 months in others.

Primary amenorrhoea
Diagnosis, investigation and management of primary amenorrhoea is discussed in Chapter 3.

The most common cause is hypogonadotropic amenorrhoea due to constitutional delay or hypothalamic dysfunction from excessive exercise, low BMI or stress.

If appropriate, depending on the cause, initiate puberty with a very low and gradually increasing dose of ethinyl oestradiol tablets or oestradiol patches, as breast and uterine growth is abnormal without gradual oestrogen exposure and low dose oestrogen contributes to normal pubertal increase in linear height. High-dose oestrogen such as that in the oral contraceptive pill (OCP) closes epiphyses, limiting final height and should not be used in the pre-pubertal population.

Secondary amenorrhoea
Secondary amenorrhoea is more common than primary amenorrhoea. The causes can be grouped into physiological and pathological (**Figure 4.1**).

The three key diagnostically useful patterns of secondary amenorrhoea are: (1) hypogonadotropic [low follicle-stimulating hormone/luteinising hormone (FSH/LH)], (2) eugonadotropic (normal FSH/LH) and (3) hypergonadotropic (high FSH/LH), as the causes and management are different. Complete serum FSH/LH and oestradiol levels as this enables you to

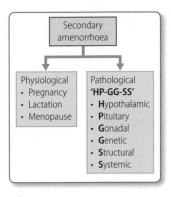

Figure 4.1 Causes of secondary amenorrhoea.

confirm the diagnostic class. Investigations then occur by possible cause within this class (**Tables 4.1** to **4.4**).

Pelvic ultrasound aids the diagnosis by providing information on the endometrial thickness, which reflects oestrogen levels, and number of follicles on the ovary (ovarian activity and polycystic ovarian morphology) and any structural abnormalities.

Good practice point

All reproductive-aged women should be considered pregnant until proven otherwise to avoid treatment with teratogens or miss the correct diagnosis. Unplanned pregnancies form around half of conceptions and many women are not aware of an early unplanned pregnancy, particularly if they also have irregular periods. The most common cause of secondary amenorrhoea is pregnancy!

Physiological amenorrhoea The key groups are tabulated in **Table 4.1**. Management is as per cause. Always perform a β-human chorionic gonadotropin (β-hCG) in secondary amenorrhoea.

Hypergonadotropic Hypergonadotropic amenorrhoea means the pituitary gland releases more FSH/LH than normal in an attempt to stimulate a poorly functioning ovary to produce oestrogen. The ovary is not able to produce oestrogen in response to these stimuli, as it has insufficient oocytes to respond. The resulting lack of negative feedback to the hypothalamus causes FSH to remain high (**Figure 4.2**).

Cause	History questions	Laboratory/Imaging finding
Physiological	• Pregnancy symptoms • Menopausal symptoms in woman over 45 years • Reports breastfeeding	• ↓FSH/LH/Oestradiol • ±↑PRL (lactation)

(FSH, follicle-stimulating hormone; LH, luteinising hormone; PRL, prolactin)

Table 4.1 Physiological causes of amenorrhoea
(FSH, follicle-stimulating hormone; GnRH, gonadotropin-releasing hormone)

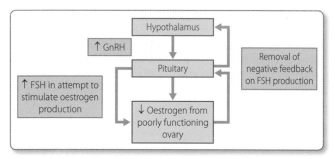

Figure 4.2 Hypergonadotropic amenorrhoea.

As follicles are responsible for ovum and oestrogen production, apart from elevated serum FSH and low serum oestradiol, a hypergonadotropic amenorrhoea will also have few ovarian follicles on ultrasound and a thin endometrial stripe.

The ovary either has intrinsically less than normal follicle amounts or has been damaged leading to ovarian failure. Causes include premature menopause [idiopathic, autoimmune and fragile X syndrome (FraX)], Turner syndrome, and following chemotherapy or pelvic radiation. In idiopathic ovarian failure, intermittent function is possible and there is a 10% lifetime pregnancy rate. For this reason, hormone replacement should include reliable contraception unless pregnancy is desired.

History Key history elements and laboratory features are tabulated in **Table 4.2**.

Cause	History questions	Laboratory/Imaging findings
Gonadal	• Symptoms of ovarian failure: Vasomotor and night sweats • RF for ovarian failure: Chemotherapy, radiotherapy and ovarian surgery	↑FSH/LH, ↓oestradiol and ↓follicles on US scan
Genetic	• Female relatives with premature menopause and male relatives with intellectual disability (FraX) • Reported short stature, webbed neck, congenital heart disease or horseshoe kidney (Turner syndrome) • Symptoms of ovarian failure as above	• ↑FSH/LH, ↓oestradiol and ↓follicles on US scan • FraX genetic test (trinucleotide expansion on FMR-X chromosome) • Abnormal karyotype 45,XO or mosaic 45,X; /46,XX

(FSH, follicle-stimulating hormone; FraX, fragile X syndrome; LH, luteinising hormone; US, ultrasound)

Table 4.2 Causes of hypergonadotropic amenorrhoea

Examination Key features include:
- Short stature, loose skin around neck, wide cubitus valgus (angle of forearm on upper arm) and cardiac murmur (in Turner syndrome)
- Genital pallor and dryness (chronic low oestrogen, in all when chronic)

Management Hypergonadotropic causes are usually permanent. Global goals of therapy for this group include providing normal adult pre-menopausal oestrogen levels with hormone replacement, screening for long-term metabolic and bone complications and fertility and family building support. The contraceptive pill is a simple hormone replacement therapy (HRT) option that is non-stigmatising and suitable if there are no other health issues such as hypertension and adult bone age has been achieved.

Specific subgroups have additional treatment goals including:
- Screening for congenital heart disease and aortic root dilatation in Turner syndrome (risk of aortic dissection) and renal

malformations (horseshoe kidney) as well as coeliac disease and hypothyroidism as these are all common
- Screening for anti-adrenal antibodies in auto-immune ovarian failure, as there is a risk of unpredictable adrenal failure which is life-threatening
- Genetic counselling for genetic causes with family screening (e.g. FraX which is associated with intellectual disability in sons of carrier women or affected men)

Eugonadotropic This includes polycystic ovarian syndrome (PCOS) and injury to the endometrium so that there is inadequate tissue growth in response to oestrogen and no menses (Asherman syndrome).

For PCOS, FSH/LH and oestradiol are in the normal range and there will be other signs of the syndrome. This usually causes oligomenorrhoea rather than complete amenorrhoea and is discussed separately below.

Table 4.3 outlines key history and investigation findings in eugonadotropic causes.

Cause	History questions	Laboratory/Imaging finding
PCOS	Symptoms of PCOS: acne, hirsutism previous irregular cycles	Eugonadotrophic. Chronic relatively stable hormones, no ovulation – no menses. Delayed bleed from thickened endometrium or fluctuation in oestrogen ↑LH, normal oestrogen, ↑androgens, +/– abnormal glucose tolerance >20 follicles per ovary on US scan +/– ↑endometrium
Structural	Repeated curettage of uterus, especially with infection (Asherman syndrome)	Normal FSH/LH/oestrogen Ovulatory mid-luteal progesterone level Normal amount of ovarian follicles and thin endometrium on US scan

Table 4.3 Eugonadotropic causes of amenorrhoea

Examination Key features on examination include acne, facial hirsutism and obesity (PCOS). Some women do not have a menstrual bleed in response to oral progesterone withdrawal (Asherman syndrome).

Management PCOS is discussed below.

Asherman syndrome is treated by operative hysteroscopy and division of adhesions with placement of short term copper intrauterine device (IUD) or small Foley catheter and oral oestrogen; however, the underlying endometrium is damaged, may not normally regenerate and if future pregnancy occurs there are high rates of abnormally adherent placentation, fetal growth restriction and risk of both manual removal of placenta, if adherent, and caesarean hysterectomy, if accreta occurs (deeper adhesion).

Hypogonadotropic In hypogonadotropic amenorrhoea, the pituitary gland is not attempting to stimulate the ovary to produce oestrogen, despite low circulating oestrogen levels.

This is abnormal and may represent an adaptive response to protect physiological reserves when the body is not capable of the additional strain of pregnancy. It is seen when physiological or psychological stress is high including in significant dieting, excessive exercise and stress.

Hyperprolactinaemia can also cause hypogonadotropic amenorrhoea, as this mimics a lactation response in the pituitary gland and suppresses release of FSH/LH. Other rare causes include Kallmann syndrome (congenital hypothalamic malformation and anosmia) and Sheehan syndrome (postpartum pituitary ischaemic injury due to hypotensive shock).

History The history in hypogonadotropic amenorrhoea is directed at identifying significant weight loss, stress, excessive exercise or symptoms or medical causes of suppressed pituitary function (**Table 4.4**).

Examination Key features include:
- Bi-temporal hemi-anopia and nipple discharge/galactorrhoea (pituitary adenoma and hyperprolactinaemia)
- Buffalo hump of fat at the back of the neck, central obesity and striae (Cushing syndrome)

Cause	History questions	Laboratory/Imaging findings
Hypothalamic	• Loss of weight (10–15%) • Stress • Exercise	• ↓FSH/LH/oestradiol • Low progesterone • Negative hCG • Thin endometrial stripe on ultrasound
Pituitary	• Anti-psychotic or metoclopramide use (prolactin) • Symptoms of prolactinoma, breast discharge, headache and bitemporal visual loss • Previous major post-partum haemorrhage (Sheehan syndrome)	• ↑Prolactin on two samples (transient rise common with exercise and nipple stimulation) • Pituitary adenoma on MRI of the brain (prolactinoma) • ↓FSH/LH/oestradiol • ±↓TSH/cortisol

Systemic	• Symptoms of significant endocrine disease:
	  – Hypothyroidism
	  – Cushing syndrome
	• Symptoms of significant general medical disease including renal failure and liver failure
		• ↓FSH/LH/oestradiol
		• ±↑TSH/↓fT4, ↑cortisol, abnormal EUC and LFT

(EUC, electrolyte, urea and creatinine; fT4, free thyroxine; FSH, follicle-stimulating hormone; hCG, human chorionic gonadotropin; LFT, liver function test; LH, luteinising hormone; MRI, magnetic resonance imaging; TSH, thyroid-stimulating hormone)

Table 4.4 Hypogonadotropic causes of amenorrhoea

- Low BMI or low body fat on skinfold testing (hypogonadotrophic due to low weight)
- Dry skin, loss of outer third of brows and hair thinning (hypothyroidism)

Management In general, hypogonadotropic causes are managed by treating the reason for central inhibition. This includes weight restoration, reducing exercise, counselling or stopping medication causing hyperprolactinaemia. Prolactinoma, a specific cause where a benign pituitary tumour produces prolactin, is either treated with prolactin-lowering medication (bromocriptine and cabergoline) or trans-sphenoidal surgery.

Metrorrhagia

Metrorrhagia refers to irregular bleeding. The most important consideration is separating irregular menses from bleeding from other lower genital tract causes, particularly inter-menstrual bleeding from the cervix, which may be erroneously attributed to menses.

Assessment

Take a detailed menstrual history and view a menstrual diary, if available. Bleeding that happens in a similar point in the cycle such as mid-cycle or pre-menstrual spotting is probably hormonal and not dangerous. Irregular bleeding is either due to anovulatory cycles (history of PCOS or risk factors common), structural pathology (e.g. polyps) or cervical pathology.

Always ask about Pap smear/cervical screening test (CST) history and risk factors for sexually transmitted infections and remember that although cervical cancer can present with irregular bleeding, chlamydia is many times more common in young adults.

Examine the cervix and vagina by speculum, take swabs for chlamydia/gonorrhoea and perform cervical screening. Request a pelvic ultrasound as this will assess for uterine causes including abnormally thick endometrium (hyperplasia) and polyps/fibroids.

> ## Guiding principle
>
> Always exclude cervical malignancy and endometrial malignancy in women with abnormal bleeding by speculum examination, co-test/smear and ultrasound (with endometrial biopsy if thickened endometrium) before treating with oral contraceptives or other medical therapy. This is because while most women with irregular bleeding do not have cancer, the minority that do will have diagnosis delayed and prognosis worsened without proper and timely assessment. Additionally, cervical cancers do present with 'menorrhagia' and lack of speculum inspection delays diagnosis.

Management

Management depends on the cause. Hormonal causes can be managed with oral contraceptives or intrauterine system

(IUS)/Mirena. Structural causes such as polyps are removed with hysteroscopically and cervicitis is treated with antibiotics. Cervical malignancy requires urgent gynaecological oncological review.

Oligomenorrhoea and polycystic ovarian syndrome

Polycystic ovarian syndrome is the most common cause of oligomenorrhoea in western societies and the most common cause of ovulatory dysfunction. This is because the rate increases with obesity and rates are high in western society.

Around 15% of adult women have PCOS. PCOS is diagnosed on Rotterdam criteria and requires two out of three criteria of:
1. Oligomenorrhoea (anovulation)
2. Clinical or laboratory support for elevated androgens
3. Polycystic ovarian morphology (PCOM) (>20 follicles per ovary)

An important caveat is exclusion of other conditions which may cause similar symptoms, in particular thyroid disorders, elevated prolactin and non-classical adrenal hyperplasia.

Good practice point

Be cautious diagnosing PCOS in adolescents as many of the features of normal adolescence overlap with PCOS. Acne is common and it is normal for young ovaries to have many follicles on ultrasound which meet polycystic ovary criteria—this is because the oocyte pool is high. Ovarian reserve, meaning the amount of follicles left to potentially ovulate, is naturally high in young women and depletes over time as new primordial oocytes cannot be formed.

Similarly, do not tell young women with PCOS they are infertile as most women do conceive with little or no assistance. Contraception is therefore, still recommended to prevent unplanned pregnancy!

Pathophysiology

Polycystic ovarian syndrome has genetic and environmental causes and there is more than one phenotype including lean/insulin resistant and obese/elevated androgens/pre-diabetic. There is an inherited predisposition, but also environmental influences from obesity and related insulin resistance. As BMI increases, the rate of PCOS increases. This is because insulin resistance causes increased androgen production from the ovaries which are then converted to oestrogens peripherally giving rise to unopposed high oestrogen, anovulation, tonically elevated LH and a higher risk of endometrial hyperplasia.

The pathophysiology is complex but abnormal ovarian androgen production, resistance to insulin and a large pool of ovarian follicles producing stable levels of oestrogen and elevated androgens underpin the clinical and biochemical findings.

History and examination

Specific clinical features of PCOS are outlined in **Table 4.5**.

Body system	Findings	Causes
Skin	• Acne • Male pattern hair (beard and chest) • Male pattern balding	Elevated androgens
Cardiovascular	↑Cardiovascular disease	Obesity, insulin resistance, elevated androgens and diabetes
Endocrine	• Impaired glucose tolerance • Diabetes	• Obesity • Insulin resistance
CNS	• Obstructive sleep apnoea • Depression and anxiety	• Obesity • Physiological stigmata of syndrome
Ovarian	Anovulation, infertility and PCOM (>20 follicles/ovary)	↑LH, ↑androgen production, lack of normal FSH/LH pattern and mid-cycle surge
Uterine	• Endometrial hyperplasia • Endometrial cancer	Anovulation and growth of endometrium under chronic oestrogen stimulation

(CNS, central nervous system; FSH, follicle-stimulating hormone; LH, luteinising hormone; PCOM, polycystic ovarian morphology)

Table 4.5 Clinical features of polycystic ovarian syndrome (PCOS)

Investigations

Key investigations in suspected PCOS seek to identify the three pillars of the Rotterdam criteria:

1. Ovulatory dysfunction
2. Elevated androgens
3. Polycystic ovarian morphology

They also screen for differential diagnoses and for complications including diabetes, impaired glucose tolerance and metabolic syndrome. These are outlined in **Table 4.6**.

Investigation	Result	Significance
Haematological investigations		
Follicle-stimulating hormone (FSH)	Normal	Eugonadotropic – excludes both hypogonadism and hypergonadism as causes of menstrual irregularity (see **Tables 4.3** and **4.4**)
Luteinising hormone (LH)	Normal or elevated	LH can be tonically elevated in PCOS however, this is not required for the diagnosis as LH is also elevated in normal women, e.g. at the time of ovulation
Cycle day 21 progesterone	Low	No ovulation
Androstenedione and testosterone	Normal or elevated	Some androgens are produced by the ovary – this is increased in PCOS
DHEAS	Normal	DHEAS elevation should prompt investigation of adrenal pathology as cause of symptoms
17-hydroxyprogesterone	Normal	Elevated in most late-onset congenital adrenal hyperplasia

Table 4.6 Key investigations in PCOS. *Continues opposite*

Investigation	Result	Significance
Prolactin and TSH	Normal	Excludes thyroid disease or hyperprolactinaemia as cause of menstrual irregularity
Anti-Müllerian hormone (AMH)	Normal or increased	Reflects increased antral follicle pool
HbA1c or OGTT	Normal or impaired glucose tolerance/ diabetes	Insulin resistance and diabetes. This may coexist with PCOS
Lipids	Elevated	Metabolic syndrome
Imaging investigations		
Pelvic US scan	• Polycystic ovaries (>20 follicles/ovary) In adult women • ±Thickened endometrium	• Increased antral follicle pool – partially recruited/matured due to dysfunctional pattern of FSH/LH release • Chronic oestrogen exposure without ovulation • Not useful in adolescents – high AFC is common

(AFC, antral follicle count; DHEAS, dehydroepiandrosterone sulphate; HbA1c, glycated haemoglobin; OGTT, oral glucose tolerance test; PCOS, polycystic ovarian syndrome; TSH, thyroid-stimulating hormone)

Table 4.6 *Continued*

Management

Management aims to address the dominant symptoms (**Table 4.5**) and identify and prevent early and late health complications (diabetes, adverse lipids, cardiovascular disease, sleep apnoea and endometrial malignancy).

Obesity In overweight women, weight control is a key component of management as this will independently improve adverse metabolic health, ovulatory dysfunction and hyperandrogenaemia.

Diet/exercise and lifestyle improvement are first-line management for this reason.

Obesity can also be treated with weight loss medications or surgery. Significantly obese younger women have the most to gain from early recourse to weight loss surgery as it is the treatment most associated with sustained long-term weight loss and reversal of metabolic complications. Diets in most women ultimately fail without long-term sustainable changes. Metformin is a common adjunct as it increases insulin sensitivity and decreases tolerance for dietary carbohydrate consumption due to gastrointestinal irritation and can improve natural ovulation rates in this population.

Elevated androgens Hirsutism (hair growth in male pattern areas such as the beard, chest and abdomen) is treated either with local therapies including depilation, laser, waxing and Vaniqa cream or with systemic anti-androgenic medications to lower the androgenic stimulation of the hair follicles, which include cyproterone acetate, finasteride and the diuretic agent spironolactone. As anti-androgenic drugs cause feminisation of a male fetus, reliable contraception is mandatory and this can be achieved in combination with oral contraception for cyproterone acetate (e.g., Dianne). Spironolactone use should also be monitored with electrolyte levels as it is a potassium-sparing diuretic.

Table 4.7 shows the pharmacological treatment of PCOS.

Acne is also treated either topically with non-hormonal drugs (benzoyl peroxide, adapalene and isotretinoin), antibiotics (tetracycline class), laser or systemically with anti-androgen drugs [usually cyproterone acetate in combined oral contraceptive pill (COCP) formulation as the oestrogen component is also helpful] or permanently with oral isotretinoin. The latter drug is a special medication and prescription is tightly controlled because reliable contraception is essential as it is highly teratogenic. It has a high long-term cure rate and is life-changing for women with severe acne.

Obstructive sleep apnoea This is a consequence of obesity and fat deposition around the airway leading to dynamic collapse

Drug	Mechanism of action
Anti-androgen	
Spironolactone	Androgen receptor (AR) antagonist, also has anti-mineralocorticoid effects and major use is as a diuretic agent
Cyproterone acetate	AR blocker, also has progestogenic effects and used in combination in COCP for this reason where anti-androgen action is desirable
Finasteride	5-alpha-reductase inhibitor prevents conversion of testosterone into active metabolite, dihydroxytestosterone
Insulin sensitiser	
Metformin	Reduction in hepatic glucose production, decreased intestinal glucose absorption and increased peripheral glucose uptake and utilisation
Topical anti-acne	
Benzoyl peroxide	Reduces sebum, decreases comedones and inhibits growth of *Cutibacterium acnes*. Resistance does not develop
Adapalene and isotretinoin	Increased epithelial differentiation and keratinisation and decreases comedones. Resistance does not develop
Tetracyline antibiotics	Lowers load of acne-forming bacteria and anti-inflammatory effect. Resistance develops
Oral anti-acne	
Tetracycline antibiotics	Lowers load of acne-forming bacteria and anti-inflammatory effect. Resistance develops
Oral contraceptives	Oestrogen decreases pituitary gonadotropin output and stimulation of androgen production by ovary, increases sex hormone-binding globulin which lowers testosterone by binding the active free hormone and preventing conversion to DHT and activation of AR when combined with cyproterone acetate, norgestimate, gestodene, drospirenone or desogestrel. There is additional direct anti-androgen effect by blocking 5-alpha-reductase and/or the AR
Isotretinoin	Decreases sebaceous glands and sebum production permanently
Topical depilatory	
Eflornithine	Inhibits anagen phase of hair production. Effect ceases when drug stopped
(COCP, combined oral contraceptive pill; DHT, dihydrotestosterone)	

Table 4.7 Pharmacological treatment of PCOS

at night due to supine position with neck muscle relaxation. Treatment is by weight reduction and nocturnal continuous positive airway pressure devices.

Infertility Infertility is due to anovulation which is more pronounced with increasing BMI. This is treated with oral ovulatory stimulants if first-line weight control measures fail and after exclusion of diabetes and other sub-fertility factors. This is because excessive weight is also associated with poor pregnancy outcomes (increased miscarriage, fetal malformation and gestational diabetes, growth disorders, pre-eclampsia, stillbirth and complicated labour) and unmanaged pre-pregnancy diabetes is independently associated with major structural malformations, in particular cardiac and neural tube with rates of 10–25% at a glycated haemoglobin (HbA1c) of over 10%.

In women who have had a normal tubal patency assessment, normal uterine cavity on ultrasound and who have a partner with a normal semen analysis, ovulation induction with either clomiphene citrate or letrozole (lower rates of twins and less unfavourable endometrial thinning) on cycle days 2–6 for up to six cycles. Counsel regarding chance of twins (10% with clomiphene citrate), ovulation rates (80% with clomiphene citrate) and pregnancy rates (cumulatively 40% with clomiphene citrate).

Refer all women who fail this and other women with multiple sub-fertility factors for fertility specialist input as they require either follicle stimulating hormone injections, intrauterine insemination or in vitro fertilisation (see Chapter 6).

Endometrial hyperplasia/malignancy Chronic anovulation and unopposed oestrogen can cause abnormal endometrial growth (hyperplasia) as progesterone which normally differentiates the endometrial cells is absent. Hyperplasia can be suspected by a history of heavy irregular periods and a thickened endometrial lining on ultrasound that often has cystic spaces. Diagnosis requires endometrial tissue for histology by either outpatient Pipelle endometrial biopsy or diagnostic hysteroscopy.

Treatment of endometrial hyperplasia is with either intrauterine (most potent) progestogen or oral progestogen for 3–6 months with repeat endometrial histology after this time to ensure the change has regressed. If complex cellular atypia is present on histology, offer hysterectomy as there is a one in

> ## Good practice point
>
> Whenever you suspect malignant or pre-malignant pathology, a tissue diagnosis is critical before referral to either an oncology service for care or management.
>
> The axiom 'when tumour is the rumour, then tissue is the issue' helps you not to forget this basic point!

three chances of associated endometrial cancer. Endometrial cancer on histology is referred to a gynaecological oncologist for staging hysterectomy as this also includes removal of sites of possible metastasis (ovaries, lymph nodes) and sampling of pelvic lymph nodes. Surgery in a dedicated cancer unit improves survival rates (see Chapter 9). Women who have not completed childbearing with atypia or cancer require individualised care in a cancer unit, conservative medical treatment is possible but relapse rates are high and pregnancy rates are low.

Cardiovascular disease Treatment of cardiovascular disease is by standard primary prevention methods if no history of events and secondary prevention methods otherwise if myocardial infarction, cerebrovascular or peripheral vascular disease occurs. Check glucose tolerance, lipid profile and blood pressure according to local guidelines. Primary prevention is with lifestyle modification of weight, exercise, diet and smoking; second line pharmacotherapy with medications including aspirin, statins and anti-hypertensives; secondary prevention uses similar methods, but has tighter treatment targets.

Menorrhagia
Menorrhagia is defined as bleeding of >80 mL per menstrual cycle; however, this is not a practical definition as menstrual loss cannot be measured accurately outside of clinical trials. Surrogate markers with good positive predictive value include

Good practice point

If a woman has iron deficiency anaemia but does not have menorrhagia, always exclude dietary factors (vegetarian), malabsorption (especially coeliac disease) and gastrointestinal loss (inflammatory bowel disease and colorectal cancer).

The same proviso applies to women with heavy periods who fail to correct their iron stores with adequate treatment. It is always safest in medicine to actively exclude rare serious pathologies rather than assume a less serious, common pathology is responsible.

Suspicious personalities make for good clinicians!

accidents/flooding, changing protection at night, iron deficiency and especially iron deficiency anaemia.

The two main groups of causes are functional and structural. Functional means the uterus is anatomically normal but heavy loss occurs and structural means the uterus has an anatomical reason for heavy bleeding.

Functional problems occur in young women and at peri-menopause. Structural problems predominate in late reproductive years and peri-menopause. Treatment is different for these groups with the former favouring medical therapy and the latter surgical therapy. This is because structural pathology can be removed and younger women are yet to complete childbearing.

Assessment

Take a history of weight, symptoms of hypothyroidism (fatigue, cold intolerance, weight gain, dry coarse skin and hair loss), irregular cycles (likely anovulation), bleeding post-surgery or dental work, paetechial rash (thrombocytopaenia), presence of intrauterine contraceptive device (IUCD), anti-coagulant medications, mass symptoms (urinary frequency and pressure from fibroids) and investigate as below.

Examine generally for pallor and tachycardia (anaemia), abdominally for a mass (fibroids) and speculum for cervical pathology and bimanual for uterine size.

Initial investigations and their utility are tabulated in **Table 4.8**.

Functional causes and management

The most common groups with functional menorrhagia are adolescents who are establishing their cycles and women in

Investigation	Utility
FBE	• Identify anaemia from iron deficiency and strongly predictive of true menorrhagia • Thrombocytopaenia if acquired coagulopathy (e.g. ITP – rare)
Coagulation studies – INR and APTT	Identify coagulation disorder (e.g. vitamin K deficiency bleeding or due to liver disease)
von Willebrand screen*	In adolescents with profuse menorrhagia or bleeding haemorrhagic ovarian cyst without history of prior successful haemostatic challenge (injury or surgery), higher risk of underlying vWD (1% of population overall)
Thyroid function tests*	Identify hypothyroidism, a cause of menorrhagia
Iron studies	Identify iron deficiency from menstrual loss
Cycle day 21 progesterone*	Identify anovulation where irregular cycles exist
STI screen – swabs or urine*	Identify menorrhagia as a consequence of endometritis
CST	Rule out mis-attributed cervical cause (cancer, rare but serious)
Pelvic ultrasound	Identify structural contributors – polyps, fibroids, adenomyosis, large uterus and assess endometrial thickness (risk of hyperplasia). Thickness >16 mm is generally abnormal
Endometrial biopsy*	Identify complex hyperplasia and malignancy

*Selective test use where history suggestive.
(APTT, activated partial thromboplastin time; CST, cervical screening test; FBE, full blood examination; INR, international normalised ratio; ITP, immune thrombocytopaenic purpura; STI, sexually transmitted infection; vWD, von Willebrand disease)

Table 4.8 Investigation of menorrhagia

peri-menopause, both of whom ovulate irregularly and have heavy irregular bleeding due to endometrial build-up from unopposed oestrogen, as discussed in PCOS above.

The next group of causes of heavy menstrual bleeding in the absence of structural uterine pathology are general medical disease (renal, liver and other), obesity (high oestrogen), thyroid disease (hypothyroidism causes anovulation), inherited or acquired bleeding disorders, use of copper IUCD and anti-coagulation.

Endometrial hyperplasia and malignancy are usually the result of chronic anovulation and the chronically anovulatory group should always have hyperplasia and malignancy actively excluded with endometrial biopsy for this reason. Women at highest risk are those who fail to respond to medical therapy, have a sonographic thickened endometrium or are over 45 years with persistent abnormal bleeding. Delay in diagnosis increases the chance of progression to malignancy.

Options for treatment of menorrhagia are:
- Conservative (containment/cups/pads)
- *Medical*:
    - Non-hormonal (tranexamic acid or iron supplements)
    - Hormonal (oral/intramuscular/intrauterine)
- *Surgical*:
    - Minimally invasive/intrauterine (myomectomy, polypectomy and ablation)
    - Definitive (abdominal, vaginal or laparoscopic hysterectomy)

The only groups who are solely recommended definitive treatment are those with cancer who require a staging procedure to attempt cure of their disease.

Management by cause is tabulated in **Table 4.9**.

Structural causes and management

Uterine intracavity structural pathology is more common in older women and rare in younger women, as older women have had more time to develop both fibroids and endometrial polyps.

Structural pathology causes menorrhagia, as the endometrial lining is distorted both by increased surface area and the distorting structure, making the overlying endometrium unstable. The most common examples are endometrial

Cause	Options
Medical disease (thyroid, other endocrine and obesity)	• Optimise underlying disease as first line • Suppress/Skip menstruation with COCP, intra-uterine system or progesterone (caution in liver disease, progesterone is hepatically metabolised) • Tranexamic acid and NSAIDs to reduce menstrual loss • Offer endometrial ablation where childbearing complete and reliable contraception (ideally tubal ligation) • Offer hysterectomy if fit for surgery and fails or declines or is not suitable for other options
Hypothyroidism	Treat with levothyroxine, cycles should improve
Irregular cycles/ anovulation	• Treat precipitant • Suppress/Skip/Control menstruation with COCP or intrauterine system • Cyclic progesterone to induce withdrawal bleeds which should be lighter as more regular
Copper intrauterine device	• Remove or change to progesterone intrauterine system • Tranexamic acid and NSAIDs to reduce menstrual loss
Anti-coagulant medication	• Cease if feasible • Insert intrauterine system • OCP is generally contraindicated and use systemic progesterone with caution (particularly Depo-Provera) • Endometrial ablation where childbearing complete and reliable contraception (ideally tubal ligation) • Hysterectomy if fit for surgery and fails or declines or is not suitable for other options. This will need peri-operative anti-coagulation plan
Inherited/Acquired bleeding disorder	• Treat if specific therapy exists (steroids, DDAVP and other) • COCP • Intrauterine system • Avoid anti-platelet medications (NSAIDs) • Ablation as above • Avoid hysterectomy unless no other option – surgical bleeding/haemostasis management complex

Table 4.9 Management options for menorrhagia. *Continues overleaf*

Cause	Options
Idiopathic (usually adolescents)	• Tranexamic acid and NSAIDs for prostaglandin inhibition to reduce menstrual loss • COCP, aim tricycle or menstrually signalled to minimise menses • Intrauterine system • Depo-Provera – will take 12/12 for 50% amenorrhoea rate and 24/12 for 75% amenorrhoea rate and irregular atrophic bleeding is common earlier
Endometrial hyperplasia and malignancy	• This is an uncommon but important group. Ensure this had been excluded, if risk factors are present • Simple hyperplasia is treated with oral or intra-uterine progesterone for 3–6 months and repeat endometrial biopsy. Risk of developing malignancy is low (1%) • Complex hyperplasia is treated with hysterectomy if childbearing is complete as one-third will have occult malignancy and intrauterine progestogen ± oral progestogen with repeat endometrial biopsy in 3 months if childbearing is not complete • Endometrial cancer should be referred for a staging hysterectomy in a cancer unit

(COCP, combined oral contraceptive pill; DDAVP, desmopressin; NSAIDs, non-steroidal anti-inflammatory drugs)

Table 4.9 *Continued*

polyps and sub-mucous (under the endometrium) fibroids, fibroids which do not distort the endometrium or cause gross enlargement of the uterus generally do not cause menorrhagia. **Figure 4.3** demonstrates the main types of fibroids (sub-serosal, intramural and sub-mucous) and endometrial polyps (sessile and pedunculated).

Structural causes are best treated surgically, as removal addresses the cause of abnormal bleeding. The two main decisions are between minimally invasive (hysteroscopic) procedures and definitive major surgical (hysterectomy) procedures. In general, hysteroscopic procedures involve minimal downtime and are preferred by most women; however, some

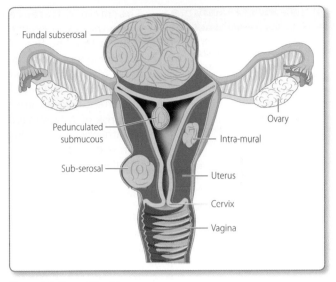

Figure 4.3 Types of fibroid.

women who have other pathology that require surgery on the uterus or those who elect for major surgery or have had prior treatment failure or recurrence will elect for a definitive solution with hysterectomy.

Hysteroscopic (intracavity) procedures Intrauterine pathology is accessed as a hysteroscopic procedure where a small camera is threaded through the cervix into the uterus. This is usually under general anaesthetic and the uterine cavity is distended with saline for visualisation.

The three main methods for resection in common use include blind manual removal with polyp forceps or under vision with an operative hysteroscope (using bipolar energy in a glycine medium) and with patented systems for specific pathologies such as the MyoSure.

As polyp forceps are used blindly, they require considerable skill and kinesthetic familiarity to avoid complication including uterine perforation and visceral injury.

Good practice point

Uterine perforations are surprisingly common in gynaecologic surgery. Most do not cause harm and heal naturally as long as the device which has made the hole is small, suction was not used, bipolar energy was not used and tissue has not been pulled out of the uterus. If any of these have occurred, do not remove the instrument as it serves as a guide to the site of possible injury in the abdomen and perform an immediate laparoscopy to assess for organ (usually bowel) injury.

It is important to ensure an experienced surgeon 'runs' the entire bowel, as small bowel injury in particular is easily missed as it will be flipped above the pelvic cavity and out of view in a standard gynaecologic laparoscopy.

The main difference between the two operative options is that the use of bipolar or monopolar energy requires glycine to distend the cavity, as saline will dissipate current. Glycine carries a small risk of symptomatic hyponatraemia and for this reason is only done where appropriate equipment exists for measuring the ongoing glycine deficit.

Hysterectomy (definitive) procedures Hysterectomy is the only procedure which is guaranteed to cure menorrhagia and is suitable for women who have completed childbearing and have failed or declined minimally invasive options.

It is major surgery and carries associated risks including bleeding, infection (wound, urine and other), venous thromboembolism (VTE), injury to other organs (bladder and ureters in particular) as well as the less often considered adhesion formation, more complex subsequent surgery, earlier menopause by 1–2 years due to interference with gonadal blood supply and vault eversion/prolapse.

Hysterectomy is performed in three ways (**Figure 4.4**):
1. Abdominally
2. Minimally invasively (laparoscopically)
3. Vaginally

The indications and contraindications for each method are described in **Table 4.10**. Either vaginal or laparoscopic procedures are preferred as they have lower complications and faster recovery than abdominal hysterectomy but these are not always possible for surgeon, equipment and patient factors (presence of prolapse or size of the uterus).

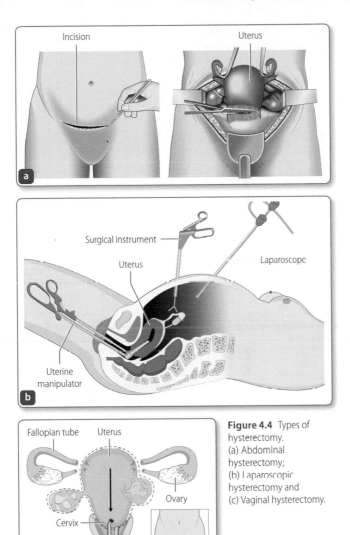

Figure 4.4 Types of hysterectomy. (a) Abdominal hysterectomy; (b) Laparoscopic hysterectomy and (c) Vaginal hysterectomy.

Method	Considerations	Indications	Contraindications
Abdominal	Pfannenstiel (bikini line cut) laparotomy Or Mid-line (vertical cut) laparotomy	• Uterus larger than 12–14 weeks size • Large fibroids • Clinician or site inability for laparoscopic procedure • Lack of prolapse/vaginal descent (nulliparity or previous caesarean)	Suitability for vaginal or minimally invasive method
Vaginal	Uterus removed vaginally, no external sutures. Can be combined with prolapse repair operation	• Small uterus • Degree of prolapse and ability to access uterus	• No prolapse (laparoscopic or abdominal safer) or poor access (narrow vaginal introitus) • Prior caesarean section or open myomectomy (laparoscopic safer, risk bladder adhesions/other adhesions) • Large uterus > 12–14 weeks size
Laparoscopic	4 port site incisions approximately 1 cm used to perform hysterectomy, uterus removed vaginally as too big to remove via a port and vaginal vault sutured laparoscopically	• Uterus under 12–14 weeks size and either prior uterine surgery or no/minimal prolapse • Ability to perform procedure	• Suitability for vaginal hysterectomy • Uterus >12–14 weeks size*

*In tertiary settings, larger uteruses can be removed laparoscopically; this requires vaginal or laparoscopic morcellation and carries the additional risk of dissemination of undiagnosed malignancy. There is also increased chance of bowel injury and the need to convert to laparotomy. This procedure is less common for this reason.

Table 4.10 Hysterectomy approaches, indications and contraindications

All gynaecologists receive training in vaginal and abdominal hysterectomy but in many centres, laparoscopic is not yet widely taught – this is changing with time, as laparoscopy becomes the preferred approach.

Other cycle disorders (polymenorrhoea and metrostaxis)

Other cycle disorders are less common and by and large respond to treatment for menorrhagia, the main two are polymenorrhoea which means short, frequent menstrual cycles of <21 days total length and metrostaxis which refers to ongoing menstrual bleeding which does not stop after the normal time menses should cease.

Polymenorrhoea

Polymenorrhoea is more common in peri-menopausal women. This is because the level of FSH required to stimulate the ovaries increases (due to fewer follicles) and ovulation quality is variable leading to an accelerated (shorter) follicular phase and deficient (therefore also shorter) luteal phase. Additionally, ovulation may not occur in many cycles leading to unstable anovulatory bleeding.

Good practice point

The cervix should always be removed at hysterectomy unless there is a very good reason to leave it behind.

This is because cervical stump cancers can occur, ongoing screening is required and may be forgotten, cancer diagnosis is often delayed and treatment is more complex and there are no proven benefits to retaining the cervix.

Clinical insight

Always prepare the vagina with betadine solution when setting up for a hysterectomy – the vagina is heavily colonised with bacteria and vault infections are likely otherwise. Surgical preparation solutions physically reduce bacterial burden and pre-incision antibiotics alone will not achieve control.

Also treat bacterial vaginosis pre-operatively, as this reduces vault infection rates and includes anaerobic cover with pre-incision surgical prophylaxis.

Good practice point

Do not omit contraception when treating women in later reproductive years as pregnancy can still occur.

Be sure to exclude pregnancy in older peri-menopausal women presenting with abnormal bleeding as many will have self-ceased contraception in misbelief they are no longer fertile. Fertility is low, but it is not zero.

Investigation and medical/surgical management options are the same as for menorrhagia above except that the OCP is contraindicated in women over 35 years who smoke, are obese with BMI > 35 kg/m², have diabetes or hypertension and in all women over 50 years. This is because the risk of cardiovascular and cerebrovascular events is elevated unacceptably with the addition of contraceptive dose oestrogen.

Metrostaxis

Metrostaxis is usually the consequence of chronic anovulation with shedding of overgrown endometrium and heavy bleeding. It can cause acute blood loss anaemia.

Acute treatment options	Regimen

Norethisterone	• Tapering/High dose:
	  – 30 mg daily for 3 days
	  – Reduce by 5 mg every 3 days until on 5 mg BD
	  – Maintain this dose until endometrial sampling and cycle control initiated – with LNG-IUS (Mirena) ideally
	• Non-tapering/intermediate dose:
	  – 5 mg TDS for 7 days
	  – Stop at 7 days, expect withdrawal bleed and then initiate ongoing cycle control

Medroxyprogesterone acetate	As for norethisterone above, but double the dose as half as potent
IV oestrogen (conjugate equine) or oral oestrogen	• 25 mg IM/IV • 10–20 mg PO in divided doses (with anti-emetics)
Tranexamic acid	1 g PO QID on days of heavy bleeding
Diclofenac sodium	50 mg PO TDS on days of bleeding
(BD, twice per day; IM, intramuscular; IV, intravenous; LNG-IUS, levonorgestrel-releasing intra-uterine system; PO, per oral; QID, four times per day; TDS, three times per day)	

Table 4.11 Treatment of metrostaxis

Investigate as for menorrhagia above and manage in two stages, firstly bring the acute bleed to an end with a tapering course of oral progesterone (for profuse bleeding with anaemia) and a non-tapering dose (for persistent bleeding without anaemia) (**Table 4.11**) and then control the anovulatory cycles as for polymenorrhoea.

Other causes of metrostaxis Other causes of metrostaxis are secondary to anti-coagulation and development of endometrial arteriovenous malformation (AVM). These are less common and the clinical history will suggest the diagnosis with clinical indication for anti-coagulation (stroke, myocardial infarction, VTE and atrial fibrillation) in the former and risk factor for AVM in the latter (surgical procedure involving endometrial curettage for miscarriage and retained placental tissue of products of conception).

Arteriovenous malformation is very rare but is important to suspect as curettage/endometrial sampling can cause profuse bleeding necessitating hysterectomy. Refer for tertiary care.

Pre-menstrual syndrome

Pre-menstrual syndrome (PMS) is defined as a constellation of mood, appetite, activity and physical changes that occur before menses and are relieved with menses. PMS is very common affecting most women to varying degrees and is not harmful. It is different to pre-menstrual dysphoric

> ### Clinical insight
>
> As metrostaxis is a symptom of anovulation, it is also a risk factor for endometrial hyperplasia. All women over 45 years with metrostaxis should have endometrial sampling to exclude this.

> ### Clinical insight
>
> Endometrial sampling should always occur prior to any treatment for menorrhagia. This is especially important in women who are planned to have an endometrial ablation or hysterectomy, as the finding of endometrial cancer may significantly change their treatment course.
>
> Permanent contraception is mandatory in women having endometrial ablation, as pregnancy is permanently contraindicated after this procedure as it is associated with high rates of severe maternal and fetal morbidity including death from placenta accreta.

Domain	Changes
Mood	• Low mood • Irritability and anxiety
Appetite	• Increased, especially for fatty- and carbohydrate-rich food
Activity	• Reduced and sleep patterns increased
Physical	• *Skin*: Oily and acne/breakouts • *Hair*: Oily • *Breasts*: Larger and tender, especially areolae • *Abdomen*: Bloating due to slow transit and relaxation of bowel and distension with gaseous contents

Table 4.12 Features of pre-menstrual syndrome (PMS)

disorder (PMDD), as this condition is associated with mood changes severe enough to cause negative effects on health, well-being and function.

The features of PMS are generally accepted to be caused by progesterone and are tabulated in **Table 4.12**.

Most women do not require treatment, of those that request it, cycle control with the contraceptive pill to provide steady low levels of progesterone rather than high luteal phase progesterone or use of IUS (Mirena) to lighten menses is often helpful, the latter because PMS is more bearable without a menses following!

Alternate options are generally reserved for PMDD and include luteal phase selective-serotonin reuptake inhibitor or in severe cases pituitary-hypothalamic-ovarian axis abolition with gonadotropin-releasing hormone (GnRH) (Zoladex) or oophorectomy and add-back HRT. This is rare.

4.4 Pelvic pain

Pelvic pain is defined as pain attributed to the pelvis and is called chronic if present for >3 months. It is very common. This definition is broad and encompasses a wide range of diagnoses including muscular, skeletal, gastrointestinal, neurologic/neuropathic, vascular, gynaecological, urologic and psychological causes.

Acute pain is caused by injury to skin, nerves, muscles bones, tendons or organs. Dysmenorrhoea from prostaglandin induced uterine contractions and transient ischaemia with menses and acute severe pain with vomiting from ovarian torsion are both gynaecological examples of acute pelvic pain.

Chronic pain involves nerve and brain changes, which result in the transmission of pain signals without tissue damage (neuropathic pain) and abnormal adaptive brain response to nerve signals which should be perceived as non-painful (central wind up). Vulvodynia, where touching of structurally normal vulval skin evokes burning pain is an example of a gynaecological chronic pelvic pain condition, as is pain postadequate surgical treatment of endometriosis despite the absence of ongoing structural pathology. Both of these conditions are a consequence of neurological change, not tissue harm.

It is more acceptable and perceived as easier to remove an organ with surgery than address chronic pain with psychological therapy, pain modulating medications, physical therapy for pelvic floor spasm and other treatments but the latter treatments are more effective.

Due to misattribution and lack of understanding of mechanism of chronic pain, women often first seek gynaecological care with chronic pelvic pain, although the cause is often not purely gynaecological and requires a multi-disciplinary chronic pain approach.

Good practise point

Chronic pelvic pain is best managed in a multidisciplinary setting, involving a psychologist, physiotherapist, gynaecologist and pain specialist with the addition (where needed) of a vascular surgeon, colorectal surgeon, gastroenterologist, neurologist and other specialists.

Clinical insight

Never attribute a women reporting pelvic pain to psychiatric or attention seeking causes until you have carefully considered and excluded all reasonable diagnoses and have considered laparoscopy to exclude superficial endometriosis, pelvic inflammatory disease and adhesive disease.

Also consider the possibility of abuse and non-consensual sexual activity in young women and girls as they are more prone to somatisation and less likely to volunteer harmful experiences.

For this reason, when assessing pelvic pain you must think outside injury to the uterus, fallopian tubes, ovaries and vagina so the correct diagnosis is made, and effective management applied.

This section discusses firstly gynaecological causes of pelvic pain and secondly a more general approach to chronic pelvic pain.

Dysmenorrhoea

Definition

Dysmenorrhoea refers to pain with menses. The experience is almost universal, but the timing has a bimodal distribution being common in adolescents (called primary) and women in late reproductive transition and less common in between.

Dysmenorrhoea is termed secondary if it develops after previously non-painful menses. Primary dysmenorrhoea is usually not associated with structural pathology and improves with age, whereas secondary dysmenorrhoea suggests that new structural pathology has developed, the most common causes are adenomyosis and endometriosis.

The mechanism and pathophysiology differ between the two age groups. Adolescents experience primary dysmenorrhoea as their endometrium is adept at producing high levels of prostaglandins. Prostaglandins cause heightened myometrial contractility and transient interruption of myometrial blood flow through spiral arteries, ischaemia and pain due to release of byproducts of anaerobic metabolism,

> ## Clinical insight
>
> Demographics are a helpful clue in your differential diagnosis in gynaecology.
>
> Fibroids are common in women of Afro-Caribbean descent, adenomyosis in obese older multi-para, primary dysmenorrhoea in adolescents, endometriosis in nulliparas not on oral contraceptives or IUSs, cervical neoplasia and pelvic inflammatory disease with lack of barrier contraception and smoking and endometrial malignancy with obesity and increasing age.
>
> There are many other examples.
>
> Arrange your differential in order of common/likely and then uncommon/dangerous, as this will make you both clinically rational and safe as you will investigate the most likely cause and exclude the causes that will harm your patient.

much like a cramp with running. Prostaglandin production and pain decrease with maturation and in particular, parity, although the mechanism is poorly understood.

Women in later reproductive years experience secondary dysmenorrhoea

Good practice point

As much of the pain in dysmenorrhoea is related to prostaglandins, inflammation and spasm as a result of cyclooxygenase (COX), pain relief that targets COX is particularly rational in treatment. Opiates are avoided and their use is a red flag sign for serious pelvic pathology.

due to the development of adenomyosis, where endometrial tissue grows into the myometrial layer. This also sheds with menses causing an inflammatory response to blood products and pain from distension of muscle fibres.

Endometriosis is the other main cause of secondary dysmenorrhoea and typically occurs after the time of primary dysmenorrhoea, as it takes time for ectopic endometrial implants to form from retrograde menses and cause inflammation, fibrosis, nerve growth and pain. Endometriosis as a new diagnosis is rare in women over 45 years, while adenomyosis is common (**Figure 4.5**). Both often co-exist.

Dysmenorrhoea which is not disabling (causing loss of attendance at school or work) and that is either not treated or requires occasional non-steroidal anti-inflammatory drugs,

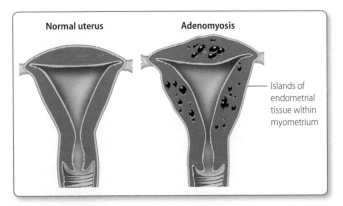

Figure 4.5 Adenomyosis.

is considered acceptable and physiological in the absence of other signs or symptoms of pelvic pathology, particularly endometriosis.

Other dysmenorrhoea should always be investigated and gynaecological pain should not be dismissed.

History and examination

Take a focussed history and examination on the features that can discriminate between diagnoses (**Table 4.13**). Bear in mind that there are exceptions to these rules.

Demographic features			Associated cause
	Age	• Adolescent	• Primary dysmenorrhoea
			• Endometriosis
		• Middle reproductive years	
		• Late reproductive years	• Adenomyosis
	Parity	• Nulliparous	• Endometriosis
		• Multiparous	• Adenomyosis
	BMI	• Normal	
		• Raised	Adenomyosis
Clinical features			
	Contraception/ Cycle control	• Hormonal	
		• Non-hormonal	Endometriosis
	Timing	Primary	Primary dysmenorrhoea
		Secondary	• Endometriosis
			• Adenomyosis
	Associated features	Deep dyspareunia and dyschezia	Endometriosis
		NSAID response	Primary dysmenorrhoea
		Menorrhagia	Adenomyosis (endometriosis)

Table 4.13 Features of dysmenorrhoea. *Continues opposite*

Demographic features			Associated cause
Examination features			
	Abdominal	Usually non-discriminatory	
	Bimanual pelvic	Enlarged tender uterus	Adenomyosis
		Nodular tender utero-sacral ligament	Endometriosis
		• Mobile • Immobile • Retroversion	• Primary dysmenorrhoea • Endometriosis
	Other	Cervical motion tenderness, cervical contact bleeding and discharge	Pelvic inflammatory disease more likely
Useful tips			
	Quality of life	• Not affected • Affected	Possible with all
(BMI, body mass index; NSAID, non-steroidal anti-inflammatory drug)			

Table 4.13 *Continued*

Investigations

Perform baseline investigations to assess for structural pathology, infection and differential diagnoses. This includes a pelvic ultrasound in all women (advise the woman to present with a full bladder as this acts as an acoustic window to visualise the uterus). Screening for sexually transmitted infections in sexually active women is also recommended but few other tests are helpful in firstline investigation of dysmenorrhoea.

Management

Management of dysmenorrhoea depends on the suspected cause, age and presence of structural pathology.

Those who have history, examination or US findings suspicious for endometriosis should be offered a laparoscopy to

Good practice point

Although it is tempting to offer a laparoscopy for all women with dysmenorrhoea to rule out superficial endometriosis, there is a small but real inherent risk of major complication and early treatment of superficial lesions which are not visible on ultrasound does not alter the natural history of the disease nor does it ameliorate the need for adjunctive medical therapy.

For this reason unless a quality women's imaging scan or examination suspects endometriosis it is reasonable to offer firstline medical therapy and reserve surgery for those with abnormal imaging, severe symptoms or who decline or are not suited for medical therapy.

Good practice point

Not all US scans are created equal. A dedicated endometriosis scan at a women's imaging provider by a suitably qualified subspecialist (called a 'COGU' scan in Au) will detect nearly all deep infiltrating/anatomy distorting endometriosis and also locate bowel involvement and adhesions. This requires very specialised training.

This is very helpful when significant endometriosis is suspected, as it allows for operative planning and increases the chance of a single complete operation at the best surgical site, for example, with a bowel and endometriosis surgeon where bowel nodules are identified.

both confirm the diagnosis and treat the endometriosis ideally with excision as this is more effective for deeper nodules than ablation and provides histological confirmation.

Those with normal scans should be offered medical therapy to achieve amenorrhoea, or as close as possible. If they have already failed medical treatment, laparoscopy is offered. The two main medical therapy options aim to create an environment of stable, high progesterone or stable, low oestrogen and progesterone. Both of these environments avoid retrograde menstruation and growth of existing implants with menses as ectopic endometrial tissue also menstruates and the inflammatory response to blood is painful.

High progesterone strategies are less harmful and better tolerated as they avoid risks of low oestrogen which include menopausal vasomotor and mood symptoms and osteoporosis and are most simply achieved with either continuous or menstrually signalled high dose progestogen OCP or a Mirena IUS.

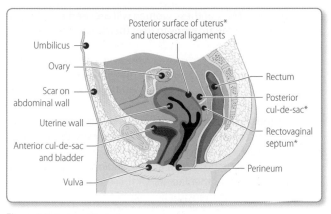

Figure 4.6 Endometriosis sites.
*Most common sites.

Endometriosis

Definition and pathophysiology

Endometriosis is defined as the presence of endometrial tissue outside of the uterus (**Figure 4.6**). In many cases, as technically both laparoscopy and histological confirmation are required to be certain, endometriosis is suspected by key history features of secondary dysmenorrhoea and deep dyspareunia and treated empirically. Severe cases will also have abnormal examination including retroversion with immobility on bimanual pelvic examination and nodular tender uterosacral ligaments. Specialised gynaecological ultrasound may detect ovarian endometriomas and

> ### Clinical insight
>
> Retrograde menstruation is a normal event in women with patent fallopian tubes and can partly explain primary dysmenorrhoea, as blood is a peritoneal irritant and its presence causes pelvic peritoneal pain.
>
> This blood naturally dissipates and is resorbed and does not lead to endometriosis in most women despite presence of a small amount of viable endometrial cells.
>
> It is not understood why some women have a peritoneal environment which allows this 'seed' to implant in ectopic 'soil' and continue to grow and shed with further menstrual cycles.

bowel nodules. Most of these women will proceed to objective confirmation with laparoscopy to treat their anatomy-distorting disease.

Not all endometriosis causes symptoms for reasons that are not well understood and up to 10% of women who have gynaecological laparoscopy for an unrelated reason will have evidence of endometriosis.

The pathophysiology of endometriosis has several hypotheses including direct implantation of retrograde menstruation through the fallopian tubes, transformation of existing peritoneal tissue into endometrial tissue as well as immunological, genetic, vascular, lymphatic and other factors. Of these, direct implantation following retrograde menstruation explains the typical location of endometriosis in the pelvis and behind the uterus and applies to most cases.

Endometriosis is divided into two types: (1) superficial and (2) deep infiltrating. This classification is useful for identifying those who will have distorted anatomy and more complex surgery but correlates less well with pain and effect on quality of life. This is because blood is effective at causing peritoneal pain regardless of the size of the endometriotic implant and endometriosis also causes surrounding nerve fibre growth and pain.

The American Society for Reproductive Medicine divides endometriosis into four stages by anatomical distribution with stage 4 representing the most extensive levels of disease. While this correlates with surgical complexity it is poorly associated with pain or quality of life.

Superficial endometriosis Superficial endometriosis means the endometriosis is visible as a vesicle, powder burn, bleb or haemorrhagic area on the peritoneum, but is not palpably thickened, nodular, hard and does not cause anatomical distortion. It is not visible on ultrasound pre-operatively.

Deep infiltrating endometriosis Deep infiltrating endometriosis (DIE) is more advanced pathology with enlarged hardened palpable nodules comprised of endometrial tissue and reactive fibrosis and scarring. This causes thickening of uterosacral ligaments and anatomical distortion with development of adhesions between the posterior uterus, ovaries, fallopian tubes and rectum and pelvic side walls. The end stage of DIE is a frozen pelvis where the rectum, uterus, ovaries and tubes are immobilised (frozen) in hard fibrotic tissue.

History and examination
Deep infiltrating endometriosis is suspected when there is either a history of prior significant endometriosis surgery and/or examination findings consistent with uterosacral ligament nodules or a frozen retroverted pelvis.

Investigation
Imaging findings vary depending on the quality of ultrasound, a women's imaging (specialist) scan will detect endometriotic nodules, obliteration of the pouch of Douglas and bowel lesions, but a non-specialist US scan will generally not have the ability to identify these findings. The presence of an endometrioma and retroversion on such a scan would be highly suggestive that DIE is present.

Management
Superficial endometriosis requires laparoscopy for diagnosis but can be treated medically (see above dysmenorrhoea section) or surgically by excision or ablation.

Deep infiltrating endometriosis is generally treated surgically by laparoscopic excision with adhesiolysis and resection of affected bowel and must have follow on medical therapy to reduce symptomatic recurrence with a Mirena to reduce menses and dysmenorrhoea. The combined OCP can also be used to suppress pain from ovarian activity. This is major laparoscopic surgery and requires careful preparation and may need to be in a combined operation with a bowel surgeon. Women who have completed childbearing are

Clinical insight

Hysterectomy (with ovarian conservation) may not cure symptoms of endometriosis, as while it originates from the uterus, microscopic peritoneal implants may not be appreciated at the time of hysterectomy. Removal of the ovaries or menopause will effectively cure endometriosis.

offered laparoscopic hysterectomy as part of their procedure as this also removes the source of future endometriotic implants and abolishes dysmenorrhoea.

Chronic pelvic pain

As outlined earlier, chronic pelvic pain involves at least 3 months of pain, has many causes in multiple systems and usually does not involve acute injury/actual tissue harm but a maladaptive peripheral sensory nerve and central response to prior stimulus. This needs careful explanation to women.

It is essential to exclude new pathology in multiple systems other than gynaecological before assigning a 'chronic pain' label. Following this, aim to treat the woman considerately and with realistic goals, avoiding harms from non-evidence-based care, inappropriate prescribing and operations. This is hard to do without input from a good psychologist and pain specialist in particular.

> ### Guiding principle
>
> A diagnostic 'label' has a powerful effect in medicine and once assigned is rarely questioned.
>
> Assign labels carefully and be certain you are correct. Many facilitate unconscious bias and can cause delay in subsequent diagnosis and it is helpful to explain to the woman both the meaning of their diagnostic label and that new pain that is different to their usual pain is just as deserving of medical care as in somebody without the pain 'label.'

History and examination

A thorough history helps to elucidate antecedent causes, the pattern and associations of pain suggest diagnoses which should be excluded before a chronic pain label is assigned and helps direct care which should always be multi-disciplinary/multi-modal.

Key features of causes are tabulated in **Table 4.14**.

Investigations

Investigations are directed to the potential cause. In most women a full blood count, inflammatory markers, pregnancy test, mid-stream urine specimen, and pelvic ultrasound are adequate and if all normal with normal examination and there

System	History	Examination
Gastrointestinal	• Bloating – fluctuates • Diarrhoea/Constipation • Blood or mucus in stool	• Resonant percussion note – gas in bowels • Often otherwise normal

Gynaecological	• Varies with menstrual cycle pattern:
	  – Worse with mid-cycle/ovulation
	  – Worse with menses
	• Prolapse pain:
	  – Aching, dragging or heavy sensation
	  – Worse at end of day
	  – Associated vaginal lump/mass
		• Signs of endometriosis:
		  – Retroversion, nodular tender utero-sacral ligaments and immobile pelvis
		• Signs of adenomyosis:
		  – Tender enlarged uterus
		• Signs of prolapse:
		  – Visible vaginal lump or bulge at introitus with Valsalva

Musculoskeletal	• Worse with movement, at end of day, better with rest • Localises poorly to pelvic floor (PF) muscles due to deep nature	• Hypertonic PF with palpable trigger points on vaginal examination • Abnormal findings on examination of lumbar spine, pelvic girdle and upper lower limb muscles by physiotherapist
Neurological	• Pain out of proportion to imaging or examination findings • Burning element common	• Normal examination • Evidence of secondary pelvic floor spasm common
Urological	• Colicky pain (ureteric) • May be loin – groin • Associated with bladder filling/emptying or voiding	• Tender bladder trigone on anterior vaginal examination • Haematuria on urine dipstick • Leucocytes/Nitrites on urine dipstick
Vascular	• Worse with prolonged standing • Aching/Heavy/Dragging nature • Associated haemorrhoids or varicose veins	Vulval, lower limb varicosities or haemorrhoids

Table 4.14 Causes of chronic pelvic pain

Intervention	Rationale
Medications: • Menstrual cycle control/minimising menstrual bleeds (continuous OCP, Mirena IUS)	• Chronic pain increases experience of acute pain and dysmenorrhoea
• Pain-modulating medications (pregabalin and tricyclic anti-depressants)	• Modulate aberrant sensory nerve adaptation causing allodynia and hyperalgesia with time can retrain normal responses • Also have pain-modulating mechanism and address central response element of maladaptive neurological chronic pain response
• Anti-depressants (tricyclic anti-depressant or selective nor-adrenaline reuptake inhibitors)	• Depression is a common association
Psychologist	Understanding that complete resolution of pain may not be achievable and teach strategies to manage with low levels of pain
Pain specialist	• Minimise poly-pharmacy • Avoid inappropriate opiate and benzodiazepine use • Centralise medication management • Can offer advanced pain options including sacral nerve stimulation implant
Physiotherapist	• Encourage and support continued physical activity, which has analgesic effect • Can treat secondary spasm and dysfunction of muscle groups including pelvic floor/levator

Table 4.15 Treatment of chronic pelvic pain. *Continues opposite*

Intervention	Rationale
Other: • Support groups • Mindfulness and lifestyle modification • Written information	• Psychologically beneficial and can provide shared tips on care • Psychologically beneficial and allow continued activity while managing pain • Access to good resource material about the nature of chronic pain, benefits of cessation of search for an organic cause and cure and rationale for chronic pain 'package' in patient-centred language are one of the most important parts of care. Without the co-operation of the woman you are caring for, this shift in mindset and approach is poorly or not accepted
(OCP, oral contraceptive pill; IUS, intrauterine system)	

Table 4.15 *Continued*

is no strong suspicion of renal stone, pelvic varicosity, inflammatory bowel disease, malignancy or disc disease, chronic pelvic pain treatment is appropriate. Laparoscopy can be considered to conclusively exclude superficial endometriosis or adhesions, but the woman should be counselled pre-procedure about the likelihood of a normal operation (negative findings) and that this is good if it occurs as it allows re-direction of care away from surgery.

The second group of women who are appropriate for chronic pain care are those with known treated gynaecological pathology who have developed chronic pain due to their condition and will not be improved by re-operation.

Management
Take a multi-modal approach as outlined in **Table 4.15**.

Genital diseases

5.1 Introduction

The genital region is composed of hair-bearing skin and mucosal tissue. The external genitalia communicate with the peritoneal cavity via the uterus and fallopian tubes. It is divided into the lower (vulva, vagina and cervix) and upper (uterus, fallopian tubes and ovaries) genital tract. This region must withstand the unique combination of challenges to integrity posed by urination, defecation, menstrual loss, sexual activity, childbearing and the transition to menopause. Additionally, the genital region can be affected by the same disease processes that affect extragenital tissue.

Genital complaints are often reluctantly disclosed by women, incompletely examined, misidentified and under-treated. The aim of this chapter is to give clinical grounding in recognising this important group of conditions and develop skills in assessing and treating them.

5.2 Clinical scenario

Presentation

A 29-year-old nulligravida attends with a 2-day history of dysuria and pelvic pain. She also reports feeling hot and sweaty and generally unwell. There are no other symptoms of note on systematic questioning. There is no other relevant medical history apart from mild asthma for which she takes Ventolin as required. Her last normal menstrual period was 4 weeks ago and she is not taking contraception, but is sexually active and has also commenced a new relationship in the last few weeks.

Examination reveals a temperature of 38.4°C, a soft non-acute abdomen (no signs of generalised peritonitis including rebound and guarding or crossed tenderness) with suprapubic tenderness, which is exquisitely tender on bimanual pelvic examination, particularly when the cervix is moved gently from side-to-side by the examiner (cervical motion tenderness). Speculum examination shows an increased abnormal discharge from the cervical os, which is mucopurulent. Urine human chorionic gonadotropin (hCG) is negative.

Diagnostic approach

The suprapubic pain, fever, cervical motion and bimanual examination tenderness all point strongly towards pelvic infection. Other possible diagnoses include urinary tract infection (UTI) and bowel pathology including appendicitis, enteritis and proctitis, but these are unlikely as neither should cause cervical motion tenderness or purulent cervical discharge.

Unprotected sexual intercourse with a new partner is an important risk factor.

Further investigations

Endocervical swabs are taken and sent for Gram stain, microscopy and culture as well as polymerase chain reaction (PCR) for chlamydia, gonorrhoea and *Mycoplasma genitalium*; these are anticipated to take a minimum of 24–48 hours to return a result but will help guide treatment later. Mid-stream urine is also sent for microscopy and culture to exclude UTI. Haematological tests show an elevated C-reactive protein and white cell count.

Pelvic ultrasound is requested to exclude a tubo-ovarian abscess, as this can require either longer treatment with intravenous antibiotics or surgical drainage.

Guiding principle

Cervical motion tenderness for pelvic organ pathology is analogous to rebound and guarding in abdominal pathology. Occasionally, severe pelvic organ pathology which has spread to involve the peritoneum as a whole presents with rebound and guarding also (e.g. ruptured ectopic pregnancy, ovarian torsion).

This is because rocking the cervix (and, therefore, moving the superior uterus) side-to-side between your fingers will place the broad ligament, which is a peritoneal fold, on tension. Like abdominal wall peritoneum/guarding, blood or pus will make this very painful and the patient may jump involuntarily, earning the term the 'chandelier sign.'

Management

A clinical diagnosis of sexually acquired pelvic inflammatory disease (PID) is made and the woman is treated with broad-spectrum intravenous antibiotics guided by local microbial resistance patterns.

She improves and is de-escalated to oral antibiotics after remaining afebrile for 24 hours. Chlamydial PCR is positive and department of health notification and contact tracing of sexual partners for the last 6 months is arranged. Reliable contraception is provided with an etonogestrel (Implanon NXT) subdermal implant before discharge home as well as the use of barrier contraception for further infection risk reduction and the woman is advised of her increased risk of ectopic pregnancy in the future.

5.3 Sexually transmitted infections

Sexually transmitted infections (STIs) encompass both local genital tract infection and blood-borne viruses, which access the circulatory system via the lower genital tract mucosa. The most common local genital infections include *Chlamydia trachomatis, Neisseria gonorrhoeae, Mycoplasma genitalium*, herpes simplex virus (HSV) and *Trichomonas vaginalis*. Common blood-borne infections include syphilis, hepatitis B and C and human immunodeficiency virus (HIV).

An understanding of common mechanisms of transmission between these diseases (sexual intercourse) is important because the common portal of entry makes co-infection frequent and logically the diagnosis of one infection equals an automatic search for the other infections.

This section deals primarily with local genital tract infections.

Good practice point

Remembering that STIs frequently occur together ensures that you will never omit blood-borne serology when a diagnosis of chlamydia or gonorrhoea is made. Similarly, advise all women on the need for contact tracing for a period of 6 months and 'safer' sex, which includes condoms on top of more reliable long-acting/reversible contraception.

Clinical insight

Any woman with a diagnosis of chlamydia or gonorrhoea should be informed of the increased chance of ectopic pregnancy in the future and informed of the need for a 6-week ultrasound to locate the pregnancy.

Genital tract STIs are responsible for significant morbidity from local effects in the lower genital tract, but can also ascend to the upper genital tract (uterus, fallopian tubes and abdomen) leading to infertility, anatomical distortion and an increased risk of ectopic pregnancy as well as PID, a serious illness which is discussed further later in this chapter. Many women will have subtle or no symptoms and for this reason, a high index of suspicion and liberal approach to diagnostic testing and empiric treatment is important.

Types

The main types of infection are bacterial (chlamydia, gonorrhoea and mycoplasma) and protozoal (trichomonas). HSV is viral.

All of these organisms with the exception of trichomonas infect the mucous membranes of the urethra, vagina, cervix, rectum, pharynx and conjunctiva and, therefore, can cause disease at multiple sites. Trichomonas infects the vagina, urethra and Bartholin's gland. Directed history taking regarding sexual behaviour is important so that the appropriate body sites are screened (mouth, vagina and anus in particular), infection detected and directed treatment commenced.

Pathophysiology and epidemiology

Genital and oral HSV are very common, affecting a large proportion of adults. There are two main types, one and two. Type one predominantly affects oral mucosa and type two predominantly affects the genital area, although there is a large degree of overlap driven by a change in societal sexual behaviours. The majority of infected people are asymptomatic or only mildly symptomatic. HSV is the most common sexually transmitted infection, but can also be non-sexually acquired through oral–oral contact or auto-inoculation.

Chlamydia trachomatis is an obligate intracellular pathogen meaning it only survives inside living cells, this makes it difficult to grow on standard culture and this is the reason PCR/nucleic acid amplification test (NAAT) is preferred for diagnosis. The incubation period is 1–6 weeks and the highest disease burden is in young sexually active adults.

Gonorrhoea is a gram-negative diplococcus and can be grown via standard culture methods; however, PCR is faster and more reliable and is recommended as the first-line test. It infects the mucous membranes and can also infect columnar epithelium. The incubation period is shorter than chlamydia at 3 days. Discharge tends to be more prominent and purulent.

Trichomonas is a protozoal infection and has an incubation period of 4–28 days.

Opportunistic screening is highly encouraged as this allows treatment of asymptomatic individuals and reduction in incidence.

Clinical features
Key clinical features of each infection are outlined in **Table 5.1**.

Diagnostic approach
Sexually transmitted infection detection is enhanced by an appropriate history that identifies risk factors, symptoms and their suspected site.

It is important to have a high index of suspicion regarding STIs as many women will not either recognise, report or have symptoms as they can be subtle and stigma is high. Change in vaginal discharge may not be noticed and dysuria and pain are often misattributed to other infections, especially urinary. Ask a sexual history in all sexually active women in particular regarding new partners, number of recent partners, sexual behaviours (vaginal, oral, anal and other), safer sex measures including condoms and do not forget to ask about especial high-risk situations such as sexual activity while intoxicated and non-consensual sex. Opportunistically, offer asymptomatic screening in women under 30 years and provide it for those who request one.

Examine symptomatic women with speculum examination to detect cervicitis (reddened, bleeding on contact and purulent discharge) and bimanual pelvic examination to detect signs of

Clinical insight

New inter-menstrual bleeding (IMB) or post-coital bleeding (PCB) in a sexually active young adult is much more likely to represent chlamydia than cervical dysplasia/malignancy.

Infections	Symptoms and signs
Chlamydia	• Frequently asymptomatic (50–70%) • Abnormal bleeding – post-coital or inter-menstrual (cervicitis) • Vaginal discharge (purulent – cervicitis and vaginitis) • Dysuria (urethral infection) • Pelvic pain
Gonorrhoea	• 50% asymptomatic • Mucopurulent vaginal discharge (gonococcal cervicitis causes more profuse discharge than chlamydial cervicitis) • Pelvic pain (25%) • Dysuria
Mycoplasma	• Increasingly recognised as a cause of cervicitis, urethritis and pelvic inflammatory disease • Often asymptomatic • Other symptoms as for chlamydia
Trichomonas	• 10–50% asymptomatic • Frothy yellow-tinged vaginal discharge or increased vaginal discharge (70%) • Vaginal itch, vaginitis and vulvitis • Dysuria • 'Strawberry cervix' can be seen in 25% (appearance from trichomonal cervicitis with punctate haemorrhages and papilliform projections)
HSV	• Painful genital vesicles on mucosal surfaces which turn into ulcers • Dysuria or acute retention from pain • Primary (first) outbreak usually the most severe • Fever
(HSV, herpes simplex virus; STIs, sexually transmitted infections)	

Table 5.1 Common STIs

complicating PID (cervical motion tenderness will be present, see PID below) and take swabs.

It is acceptable to defer a sensitive examination such as pelvic examination where no symptoms are reported unless there is another indication such as cervical screening. In these women, offer either self-collected vulvovaginal swabs or first-pass (as opposed to mid-stream) urine for PCR instead.

Investigations

Symptomatic women require a high vaginal and endocervical swabs for chlamydia/gonorrhoea/mycoplasma and trichomonas PCR. Concurrent microscopy, culture and sensitivity (MCS) swab is helpful as it can be used later to identify antibiotic sensitivities for some infections with high rates of resistance (especially gonorrhoea) and PCR will not give this information. This will directly identify STIs in the cervix.

> ### Guiding principle
>
> Sensitive history taking is a key in the areas of sexual health. Always ensure you signpost the area of questioning and the reasons for the questions as well as routinely providing reassurance regarding confidentiality and adequate privacy. Avoid such questioning in the presence of partners, family members and friends and make it your routine to interview all women on their own. This is readily accepted by nearly all support persons.
>
> Be aware of the considerable stigma around disclosing STIs as well as high-risk behaviours and keep your tone supportive and non-judgemental.

First-pass urine, which means collecting the first part of the urine stream and not the first void of the day, is able to identify STIs with slightly lower sensitivity. It is reserved for asymptomatic screening.

Principles of management

The principles of management of a confirmed STI are:
- Notify the woman
- Treat with appropriate antibiotic as guided by local antimicrobial advice
- Complete full STI screen including blood-borne viruses
- Advise contact tracing of sexual partners, usually for the preceding 6-month period
- Notify the department of health or appropriate local authority for all notifiable diseases
- Provide a test of cure no sooner than 1 month after treatment
Opportunistically complete cervical screening, vaccination and contraceptive care as these are often needed.

5.4 Pelvic inflammatory disease

Pelvic inflammatory disease is a relatively common gynaecological infection and refers to infection of the upper genital tract and abdomen usually from organisms native to or introduced to the lower genital tract. PID is important to recognise and treat promptly as it rapidly causes serious complications.

Types

Pelvic inflammatory disease has two main diagnostic groupings: (1) sexually acquired and (2) non-sexually acquired. The distinction is important as the pathogens differ and so do the optimal antibiotics to treat the infection.

Sexually-acquired PID involves infection with a sexually transmitted organism, which ascends to the upper genital tract, fallopian tubes and abdomen. Non-sexually-acquired PID develops from endogenous vaginal flora, which may be facilitated by dysbiosis (bacterial imbalance) such as bacterial vaginosis (BV) or surgical instrumentation.

Pelvic inflammatory disease causes widespread inflammatory response in the cervix, uterus, fallopian tubes and surrounding anatomy resulting in abnormal vaginal bleeding, adhesions, pyosalpinx, pelvic abscesses and chronic pain, infertility and ectopic pregnancy.

Clinical features

The key clinical features of PID can be divided into systemic and pelvic. Systemic features include fever, chills and rigors as well as right upper quadrant pain from peri-hepatic adhesions (Fitz–Hugh–Curtis syndrome) (**Figure 5.1**).

Pelvic features include offensive vaginal discharge, pain and cervical motion tenderness.

Diagnostic approach

Take a history of the above symptoms, establish severity of illness and elicit proximal risk factors. These are:

- Unprotected sexual intercourse
- Multiple sexual partners
- Previous STI
- Symptoms of STI including new PCB, vaginal discharge and dysuria
- New deep dyspareunia caused by inflammation and abscess in the pouch of Douglas

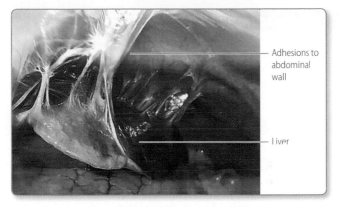

Adhesions to
abdominal
wall

Liver

Figure 5.1 Fitz–Hugh–Curtis syndrome.

- Recent gynaecological procedure (with or without known BV)

Severity is established collectively by symptoms of distributive shock (low blood pressure and fainting), sepsis (confusion/delirium, rigors, high fever > 38.5°C and reduced urine output), pelvic collection (pain and dyspareunia) and deranged electrolyte, liver function, coagulation and renal function.

Also actively question regarding other causes of septic symptoms and pelvic pain and exclude these in your investigations (below).

Guiding principle

Sepsis is a medical emergency and requires urgent treatment. This is because the sufferer is at risk of end-organ dysfunction and can die without prompt recognition and treatment. Young, healthy people will decompensate late and you will miss these cases without due care. If in doubt, always admit and treat with parenteral antibiotics.

Good practice point

Always establish the date of the last normal menstrual period and explore pregnancy status. This is because antibiotic options are different in pregnancy and an ectopic pregnancy is more likely if PID is present.

The most common diagnostic confounder is urinary sepsis, which is usually distinguishable by the presence of dysuria and urinary frequency. Less frequently, PID can be mistaken for

Good practice point

A first-void urine PCR is not ideal as a test for STI in women with symptoms of infection. This is because the test is not sampling the cervix and there is a small false-negative rate. An endocervical swab is more reliable and can also provide microscopy and culture sensitivities.

The main reason a first-void urine is used for asymptomatic community screening is because patient compliance is higher than with self-collected swabs meaning the urine test performs better in this setting as more women actually do the test.

Clinical insight

Unless the patient is in septic shock or the collection is very large, tubo-ovarian abscesses are initially managed conservatively as 75% of women respond and operating in an acutely infected pelvis increases the risk of bleeding and other complications. Delayed operation once the acute inflammation has settled is ideal, aiming for drainage rather than complete removal of the phlegmon due to morbid adhesion formation.

gastrointestinal infections, which are distinguishable by a change in bowel habit.

Investigations

Key investigations seek to confirm the diagnosis, establish severity and search for the cause (**Table 5.2**).

Management

All but the mildest of cases should be treated as an inpatient with intravenous antibiotics.

The mainstay of therapy in PID is broad-spectrum empiric antibiotics covering gram-negative, anaerobic and fastidious organisms. Patients require supportive care with analgesia, hydration and correction of metabolic derangements. It is essential to identify any tubo-ovarian abscesses or pelvic collections, as these require a prolonged course of antibiotics or surgical drainage.

Once the woman is improving and stable on oral antibiotics, outpatient management continues and repeat imaging is arranged for resolution of collections. If a sexually transmitted organism was identified, the woman should also have a 'test of cure' 1 month after treatment and be advised about the long-term risk of ectopic pregnancy and infertility.

Investigation	Indication	Reason
Haematological: • FBE and CRP	• ↑WCC/CRP in infection	• Confirm diagnosis and track response to treatment
• EUC	• Acute kidney injury in sepsis	• Identify and treat renal impairment and rehydrate. Adjust renally excreted medications
• LFT	• Sepsis-related impaired liver function and Fitz–Hugh–Curtis syndrome	• Illness severity and track response to treatment
• hCG	• Identify pregnancy	• Avoid medications that are contraindicated, search for viability and location of pregnancy
Microbial: • Endocervical or high vaginal MCS	• Identify specific organism	• Targeting of antibiotic therapy and resistance patterns
• MSU/MCS	• Exclude urinary tract infection	• Exclude differential diagnosis and treat
• Blood culture C + S	• Detect bacteraemia	• Marker of severe infection and longer duration of therapy
PCR: • High vaginal or endocervical PCR for chlamydia, gonorrhoea, trichomonas and *Mycoplasma genitalium*	• Identify specific organism	• Targeting of antibiotic therapy
Imaging: • Pelvic ultrasound • CT scan	• Identify complicated PID/abscess formation	• Alters treatment duration and follow-up. May need surgical intervention
(CRP, C-reactive protein; EUC, electrolyte, urea and creatinine; FBE, full blood examination; hCG, human chorionic gonadotropin; LFT, liver function test; MCS, microscopy, culture and sensitivity; MSU, mid-stream specimen of urine; PCR, polymerase chain reaction; PID, pelvic inflammatory disease; STI, sexually transmitted infection; WCC, white blood cell count)		

Table 5.2 Investigations in PID/STI

5.5 Common non-sexually acquired infections

There are many infections that are not sexually transmitted with a predilection for the female genital tract and these cause considerable social and economic burden. The two most common examples of non-sexually acquired infections are *Candida* and BV. Both occur due to pathological overgrowth of commensal organisms.

Candida, the most frequent infection, affects nearly all post-pubertal women at some point in their lives, causes intense itch/irritation and is relatively costly to treat in many settings.

Bacterial vaginosis is also common, causes unpleasant odour and has a high recurrence rate. Apart from nuisance factor, BV is associated with increased susceptibility to STIs and post-procedural pelvic infection.

Candida

Candida (or 'thrush') is a fungal organism with many species, the most common affecting humans is *Candida albicans*, which colonises most post-pubertal women. Nearly all will have a symptomatic episode of overgrowth resulting in clinical thrush at some point in their life.

> ### Good practice point
>
> Not all *Candida* on vaginal swab requires treatment for thrush. This is because *Candida* is a commensal and will be found on vaginal swab in many post-pubertal women. Unless the swab is performed for symptoms of thrush (primarily itch with white discharge), the presence of *Candida* can be ignored.

Candida is rare outside of menstruating women as oestrogen both facilitates *Candida* proliferation directly and provides a reduction in the ability of vaginal epithelium to resist its overgrowth.

Common precipitants can be remembered as microbial, environmental and hormonal. They include antibiotic therapy as this kills vaginal commensals and allows overgrowth (microbial). Environmental precipitants include obesity, tight non-breathable clothing, genital moisture and occlusion with frequent exercise or swimming and remaining in damp clothing.

High oestrogen levels as found with oral contraceptive use and pregnancy are hormonal risk factors.

Some women develop recurrent *Candida* infections. While diabetes is associated with recurrent candidiasis, investigation usually does not reveal a cause.

Clinical insight

In a pre-menarchal or post-menopausal woman, itch without discharge or discharge without itch is not likely to be candidiasis and a search for other causes of vulval pruritus should occur.

History and examination

This is straightforward in most cases of suspected vulvovaginal candidiasis.

Key features are vulvovaginal pruritus, pain and a curdy thick white discharge. Exclude other diagnoses that are outlined in **Table 5.3**.

The majority of adult women self-diagnose their condition and seek over-the-counter treatment.

Therefore, you are more likely to see women with a first episode, recurrent symptoms or atypical features.

The first step is to confirm the diagnosis is thrush and the second step is to confirm the reason for recurrent disease.

This requires examination, exclusion of pathological predisposing factors (diabetes and immunosuppression) and vulval/vaginal swab to exclude *Candida glabrata*, in particular, as this does not respond to azole and other common *Candida* treatments.

Investigations

Always examine the vulva and vagina by speculum, do not simply look for white discharge; diagnosis of thrush on visual inspection alone has surprisingly poor specificity, unless performed carefully for supportive features.

Normal vaginal discharge is white and can be thicker in the second half of the menstrual cycle due to the action of progesterone on cervical secretions. Candidal discharge is classically thick, clotty (described as cottage cheese like), adherent to vaginal walls and when removed exposes erythematous vaginal tissue.

Condition	History/Examination findings	Investigation
Lichen sclerosis	• Prominent itch • No discharge • Genital pallor, obliteration of labia minora and may involve anal margin • Pre-menarchal or post-menopausal	Vulvoscopy Biopsy
Vulval neoplasia	• Prominent itch • ± Visible plaque of abnormal tissue	
Pubic lice	• Prominent itch and no discharge • Presence of pubic hair • Visible mites ± bite sites with magnifying glass	Clinical diagnosis
STI (chlamydia, gonorrhoea, mycoplasma and trichomonas)	• Discharge – mucopurulent, bloody, frothy, green and yellow • Often no itch • May disclose new sexual partner	NAAT/PCR
Vulvovaginitis	• Exposure to irritants, e.g. soap, feminine hygiene products, liners and friction • Usually pre-pubertal or post-menopausal	Swabs for microscopy Biopsy rarely required
(NAAT, nucleic acid amplification test; PCR, polymerase chain reaction; STI, sexually transmitted infection)		

Table 5.3 Genital conditions

Take microscopy swabs for culture and consider swabs for PCR for STIs in women with risk factors or other pathological discharge (blood, green, yellow and frothy).

Management

Treatment is straightforward in uncomplicated cases with a course of either an 'azole' or nystatin antifungal agent. Many formulations are available and all are efficacious, the most common are the imidazoles (fluconazole) and polyenes (nystatin).

Recurrent candidiasis, if there is no addressable predisposing feature (hormonal, environmental and microbial), is treated by several methods including:

- Prolonged course of usual treatment
- Prolonged course of oral suppressive treatment, e.g. for 1–3 months
- Intermittent suppressive therapy with oral fluconazole, e.g. for 1 week a month in the luteal phase (most likely time of symptoms)
- Treatment of sexual partners

There is no superior option and despite these measures, recurrence rates are high. This is because eradication is not possible and affected women have a predisposition to *Candida* overgrowth.

Candida glabrata is treated with intra-vaginal boric acid pessaries; these are available through compounding pharmacies.

Candidiasis is very uncommon in pre-menarchal and post-menopausal women as the growth of *Candida* requires estrogenisation of the vagina and vulva and genital pruritus and irritation are relatively non-specific symptoms. In these groups, overgrowth is particularly rare without a further pre-disposing factor such as diabetes or immunosuppression or prolonged nappy wearing. Vulvovaginitis is often from other causes and *Candida* treatment should not be initiated without exclusion of these and a positive vulval swab for *Candida* for this reason.

In these atypical groups, if you confirm thrush, exclude immunosuppression and diabetes, when clinically appropriate. In older women, exclude vulval dermatoses such as lichen sclerosis with and vulval neoplasia with vulvoscopy and biopsy. These are distorting and premalignant conditions and require specific specialist treatment.

Bacterial vaginosis

Bacterial vaginosis is considered a dysbiosis, an overgrowth of already present gram-negative and anaerobic vaginal flora, including *Gardnerella vaginalis*. Dysbiosis is normally prevented by high numbers of hydrogen peroxide producing lactobacilli and a low vaginal pH. Disruption of lactobacilli count and loss of acidity lead to other flora flourishing and, once present, vaginal pH remains raised and biofilms form. Antibiotics penetrate biofilms poorly resulting in rapid proliferation after antibiotic treatment. This is the major cause for the very high recurrence rate of BV.

Antecedent risk factors include obesity, broad-spectrum antibiotic use, douching, spermicide and condom use, multiple sexual partners and a history of BV.

History and examination

In general, the diagnosis is straightforward as women report an unpleasant fishy odour and thin grey-white vaginal discharge. The odour is worse after intercourse as semen is alkaline and releases amines from the discharge. It is worthwhile enquiring about modifiable behavioural risk factors (in particular douching) as this permits education about helpful behaviour change.

Mild vulvovaginal irritation can occur, but significant dyspareunia or pain suggests another diagnosis.

Examination is generally also straightforward and is normal apart from grey-white vaginal discharge adherent to vaginal walls with a fishy odour.

Investigations

Take vaginal swabs for both MCS and also PCR for chlamydia, gonorrhoea and trichomonas as STIs also cause abnormal vaginal discharge. A saline 'wet preparation' on a slide for microscopy is helpful, if available.

Microscopy from a vaginal swab will show a Gram stain with clue cells, vaginal pH will also be >4.5 and 'whiff' test positive for odour; these three items plus characteristic discharge form Amsel's criteria for the diagnosis of BV.

Only three are required to make the diagnosis.

Of all the findings, clue cells are the most specific for BV.

Management

Asymptomatic women do not require treatment unless they are pregnant (as there is an association with preterm birth and miscarriage) or having gynaecological procedures (risk of pelvic infection is increased).

Treatment is by addressing antecedent factors where possible, particularly for spermicides and douching. Topical or systemic antibiotics that cover anaerobes, such as metronidazole or clindamycin, are the mainstay of treatment, with a biofilm inhibitor (Fleurstat) being added for resistant or recurrent cases.

Maintenance courses can help to prevent relapse. Probiotic consumption is also helpful and if vaginal lactobacilli preparations are available, these are also helpful.

5.6 Lichen sclerosis and other vulvar dermatoses

The genital skin is as prone to dermatological conditions as the skin of other parts of the body; however, diagnosis is often delayed as women are often reluctant to disclose genital symptoms and present when these are severe.

Do not forget to ask about symptoms of genital dermatoses, which include pain, itch, changes

Good practice point

Lichen sclerosis is often diagnosed when considerable anatomic distortion is present and this is irreversible. A good gynaecological history habit includes enquiry for symptoms of itch, pain and skin changes. Part of a routine 'well-woman-screen' should include questions about contraception/safer sex, breast self-examination/screening, cervical screening and vulval awareness including self-inspection with a mirror, if concerns develop.

to anatomy and in vulval skin and always inspect the vulva before speculum examination, this will reduce the chance of missing vulval pathology. Women with non-vulval skin problems should be asked about control and if their vulva has been involved previously.

One format for a comprehensive-focussed gynaecological history is shown below:

- *Pain and bleeding*: Dysmenorrhoea, dyspareunia, pelvic pain, menses, IMB and PCB and date of last menstrual period (LMP)
- *Fertility and contraception*: Desire for pregnancy, prior fertility problems, current contraception and satisfaction and prior methods
- *Prolapse and incontinence*: Prolapse symptoms, mass, urinary bowel, coital, urinary incontinence, stress and urgency and frequency of accidents
- *Pruritus and discharge*: Itch, abnormal discharge and prior STI and non-STI
- *Well-woman check*: Breast self-examination/screening, cervical screening, sexual and domestic safety and vulval awareness

The most common vulval dermatoses you will encounter are atrophic vulvovaginitis, lichen sclerosis, general dermatitis and lichen simplex, infective conditions and occasionally vulval neoplasia.

Other diagnoses are possible including lichen planus, vulval psoriasis, vulval Paget's disease, squamous and basal carcinomas, melanoma, drug eruption and many others. These are uncommon and specialised. The early practitioner is expected to recognise when a presentation is different to the common conditions above and refer to a specialised vulval clinic or for a dermatology opinion.

These conditions, key features, diagnosis and management are tabulated below in **Table 5.4**.

Avoid prescribing long-term moderately potent or potent steroids without biopsy to confirm your diagnosis. This is because misdiagnosis of high-grade vulval neoplasia or early

Condition	Symptoms/Cause	Signs	Diagnosis	Management
Atrophic vulvovaginitis	• Vaginal dryness • Dyspareunia • Light post-coital bleeding • Post-menopause	• Labia minora and vaginal pallor • Dry appearance • Petechial bleeding inside vaginal walls on pressure/speculum examination	• Clinical examination and supportive history	• Vaginal oestrogen cream • Vaginal lubricant
Lichen sclerosis	• Vulval anatomy change – shrinking of minora and narrowing of introitus • Dyspareunia • Itch – usually prominent	• White pal or in 'figure of eight' distribution around minora and anus • Absence of minora – resorbed by disease • Narrowed introitus • Vagina normal above	• Vulvoscopy and biopsy • Usually also clinically apparent	• Moderately potent topical steroid + topical oestrogen • Biannual vulval gynaecological review (risk of vulval neoplasia) • Vulval self-inspection monthly
General dermatitis and lichen simplex	• Exposure to pad, liners, soaps and hygiene products • Chronic scratching	• Erythema and excoriation ± lichenification (thickened rough appearance) • ± Signs of superimposed infection	• Clinical history + Examination usually adequate • Biopsy in cases that fail to respond to treatment	• Remove irritant • Antihistamine and gloves at night • Vulval care habits (no soap, cotton underwear, underwear free time, avoidance of occlusion and simple emollients) • ± Short course steroid and antibiotic

Table 5.4 Management of common vulval complaints. *Continues overleaf*

Condition	Symptoms/Cause	Signs	Diagnosis	Management
Infective conditions	• *Molloscum contagiosum*	• Papules with a central dimple • Often on extragenital skin • Affected household contacts	• Clinical	• Time, Aldara cream, local destructive procedures – immune response clears infection once develops
	• Warts/Condylomata	• Cauliflower or flat frond-like lesions		
	• Herpes simplex	• Painful groups of vesicles and shallow ulcers	• Clinical and PCR swab from ulcer or vesicle	• Oral antiviral therapy and analgesia
	• Chancre (primary syphilis)	• Painless papule	• Clinical ± Dark field microscopy from swab of lesion ± PCR from lesion ± Positive serology	• Benzathine penicillin
Vulval neoplasia	Itch, ± plaque, presence of HPV infection or chronic vulval dermatosis (e.g. lichen planus)	• Acetowhite on vulvoscopy • May have visible plaque	• Vulvoscopy and biopsy • Colposcopy in HPV-positive cases as risk of cervical neoplasia	• Excision of high-grade disease. • Vaginal oestrogen • Topical imiquimod, 5-FU or laser in specialized settings

(5-FU, 5-fluorouracil; HPV, human papillomavirus; PCR, polymerase chain reaction)

Table 5.4 *Continued*

malignancy will worsen prognosis and delay appropriate care. Additionally, the small risk of steroid side effects from topical vulval use is warranted only when you are certain of the correct diagnosis.

Reproduction

6.1 Introduction

Gynaecology covers the entire span of a woman's lifetime. One of the most important times of a woman's life are her 'reproductive years,' the time between menarche (when she has her first period) to the time of menopause (when she has her last period). During this time, a woman may require counselling about contraception, early pregnancy loss, termination of pregnancy, fertility and pregnancy. Women in their reproductive years are also at the highest risk of domestic and intimate partner violence.

6.2 Clinical scenario

A 35-year-old woman presents with her 40-year-old male partner with infertility. They have been having regular unprotected vaginal intercourse for 13 months without successful conception. Neither she nor her partner has ever conceived previously. The woman has regular periods, which are not painful or heavy. She has no other known medical conditions and has never had surgery. Her partner is also healthy and well and had never had any surgeries. They are both very concerned that they may not be able to have children.

Diagnostic approach

Infertility occurs in approximately 15% of the population. Causes are approximately equally distributed between partners.

Investigations aim to determine any treatable causes and are divided into male factor and female factor investigations. After focussed history and examination, the male partner is investigated with semen analysis (SA) and immunobead testing for anti-sperm antibodies. The female partner is investigated for central, ovulatory, tubal and uterine causes. Parental karyotyping can also be useful in situations where the above investigations are abnormal.

Further investigations

Semen analysis is normal and there are no anti-sperm anti-bodies. The woman has normal hormonal testing and a normal pelvic US. At laparoscopic assessment with dye studies, the woman is diagnosed with stage 4 endometriosis with bilaterally obstructed tubes.

Management

The couple is counselled regarding their options for fertility management. It is recommended that she has in vitro fertilisation (IVF) and she undergoes a standard IVF cycle. She has a fresh embryo transfer, which is unsuccessful, but successfully conceives in her subsequent frozen transfer.

6.3 Contraception

Contraception gives a woman control over her fertility choices and allows her to decide whether she wishes to have a pregnancy or remain childless and also allows her to control the timing of pregnancy. This empowerment is the reason why the United Nations have declared contraception as a human right.

Conception occurs in a specific window in the menstrual cycle and is possible for around 24 hours around the time of ovulation. The biology and viability of the egg and sperm influence this window of time. Once ovulation occurs, the oocyte survives in vivo for up to 24 hours. Sperm survive in the female genital tract up to 5 days. The most fertile time during a woman's cycle is, therefore, in the period of 5 days leading up to ovulation and 1–2 days after ovulation. Relying on this knowledge alone for contraception leads to high unintended pregnancy rates, as most women cannot time their ovulation accurately enough to be certain of avoiding their fertile window.

Pearl index

The Pearl index is used to standardise how 'well' a method of contraception performs and how it compares to other methods. It is a measure of the percentage of unintended pregnancies that occur using a contraceptive method over a year of use.

This is divided into 'perfect' use (when used correctly) and 'typical' use (usually more representative of the actual failure rate of the contraceptive method).

Natural methods

By understanding the mechanisms of ovulation and fertilisation, it is possible for a woman to have some level of control in terms of avoiding pregnancy. These methods can be effective with 'perfect use,' but are not nearly as effective as other 'artificial' methods of contraception and are unreliable. These methods are favoured by some religious groups and those who eschew medication.

Timed intercourse (billings method)

This is where intercourse is timed to be outside of the 'fertile window' discussed above. This relies on the accurate knowledge of a woman's cycle and depends heavily on cycle regularity. It has other drawbacks of permitting intercourse when the woman's biological drive is lowest and removing spontaneity.

Withdrawal

This method involves the male partner withdrawing his penis from the vagina prior to ejaculation. It depends on very accurate timing and cannot account for the small amount of sperm that may be present in pre-ejaculate, the fluid that can be released prior to ejaculation. Failure rates are high for this reason.

Short acting

Contraceptives that afford reproductive control quickly, are reversible and can be stopped easily are considered as short-term contraceptives. These include barrier methods (e.g. condoms) and hormonal methods such as the combined oral contraceptive pill (COCP). **Table 6.1** summarises the efficacy, advantages and disadvantages of these methods.

Method	Pearl index Typical (T) Perfect (P)	Advantages	Disadvantages and side effects	Non-contraceptive benefits
Male condom	15 (T) 2 (P)	• Easily reversible and quick return to fertility upon cessation • Cheap • Non-hormonal • Does not need ongoing use when not sexually active	• Removes 'spontaneity' • Must be worn incorrectly • May reduce sensation	Protects from bacterial and some viral sexually transmitted infection (STI)
Diaphragm	16 (T) 6 (P)	• Cheap • Non-hormonal • Does not need ongoing use when not sexually active • Quick return to fertility upon cessation	• Not as effective as other methods • Requires fitting • Timing of insertion is important and removes spontaneity • Needs to be left in place at least 6 hours after sex	None
Combined oral contraceptive pill	8 (T) 0.3 (P)	• Can control cycle and skip periods • Very effective with perfect use	• Needs to be taken every day • Can have a delay in return to fertility of up to 6 months • Bloating, breast tenderness and mood changes • Not suitable for women >35 years who smoke • Slightly increased thromboembolism risk	• Prevents benign ovarian cysts • Reduced risk of ovarian cancer • Improves pre-menstrual tension • Reduced menorrhagia and dysmenorrhoea

Table 6.1 Short-acting contraception. *Continues opposite*

Method	Pearl index Typical (T) Perfect (P)	Advantages	Disadvantages and side effects	Non-contraceptive benefits
Vaginal ring	8 (T) 0.3 (P)	• Do not need to take every day • Quick return to fertility upon cessation	• Expensive • Bloating, breast tenderness and mood changes • Not suitable for women >35 years who smoke • Slightly increased thromboembolism risk	None
Progesterone-only pill	8 (T) 0.3 (P)	• Does not interfere with breastfeeding • No oestrogen-related side effects • Quick return to fertility upon cessation	Needs to be taken every day at the same time (within 3 hours)	None

Table 6.1 *Continued*

Male condom

This is a sheath made from latex (although latex-free options are available) that is placed over the erect penis prior to intercourse. It is important that these are used correctly, being careful to avoid seminal contamination of the external surface of the condom. They work by mechanically preventing the entry of sperm into the uterus. They must be worn before any ejaculation has occurred. As they are an effective barrier method of contraception, they protect from many sexually transmitted infections (STIs) including chlamydia, gonorrhoea, syphilis, hepatitis and human immunodeficiency virus (HIV).

Diaphragm

This is a flexible cup (**Figure 6.1**), which is inserted into the vagina, covering the cervical opening preventing the entry of sperm into the uterus. It can be inserted by the woman herself, although it is worthwhile having them fitted professionally in the first instance. Additional spermicide is applied to the cup to enhance efficacy. These are rarely used.

Combined oral contraceptive pill

This is a very commonly used form of reversible contraception.

The COCP contains both an oestrogen and a progestogen (synthetic progesterone) and works by preventing

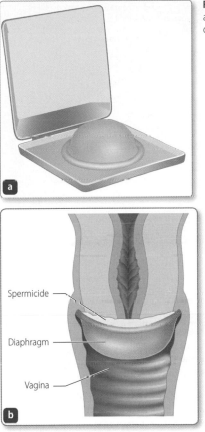

Figure 6.1 (a) Diaphragm and (b) Ideal positioning of diaphragm.

ovulation, thickening cervical mucus and thinning the endometrium. There are some forms of contraception which also include the anti-androgen, cyproterone acetate (e.g. Diane ED). These have the additional benefit of reducing signs of hyper-androgenism such as hirsutism and acne and are a good option for women with polycystic ovarian syndrome (PCOS).

Most COCPs come in 28-pill packets with 21 hormonally active pills (containing oestrogen and progesterone)

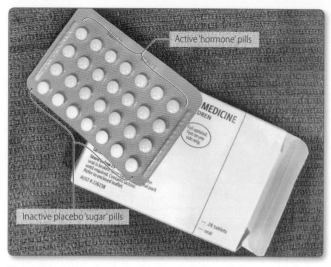

Active 'hormone' pills

MEDICINE
DREN

Inactive placebo 'sugar' pills

— 28 tablets
— oral

Figure 6.2 Combined oral contraceptive pill (COCP) pack showing the sugar and hormone pills in circuit.

Clinical insight

Menstruation is initiated by a decline in progesterone. When the placebo pills in a COCP packet are taken, the subsequent fall in progestogen stimulation results in a 'withdrawal bleed.' This is not technically a 'period,' as it is not preceded by ovulation.

and 7 placebo 'sugar' tablets (**Figure 6.2**). They are different colours for ease of identification and the pack also has a red section where the withdrawal bleed is expected – this starts around 2 days after the placebo pills as there is a lag as the synthetic oestrogen and progesterone are metabolised and levels fall until bleeding occurs.

There are two methods of commencing the COCP: (1) a 'quick start' at any point in the woman's cycle and (2) a 'traditional start', waiting for a menstrual bleed before commencing.

With a traditional start, the woman is protected from pregnancy immediately. With a quick start, the woman is protected after seven active tablets have been taken. Because of the small chance of an early pregnancy at the time of 'quick start,' the woman should be advised to perform a pregnancy test if she does not have her first withdrawal bleed at the end of the active tablets.

The woman takes one tablet per day at the same time. If she misses a pill by >24 hours, has vomiting or diarrhoea or is taking any medication that can interfere with metabolism of the COCP (e.g. rifampicin and anti-epileptics), then she needs to use alternative contraception (e.g. condoms) or remain abstinent for 7 days (while also taking the active hormonal pills each day) before she is protected from pregnancy again. When the placebo ('sugar') pills are taken, the woman will have a withdrawal bleed. Menses can be avoided by skipping the placebo pills and moving straight onto the next packet with active hormonal pills. This is very safe and has higher satisfaction and lower unintended pregnancy rates.

The COCP should not be used in women who have a contraindication to oestrogen, particularly those being treated for hormonally active cancer or those with a history of venous thromboembolism (VTE).

Vaginal ring

This is a soft plastic ring, which contains both oestrogen and progesterone and is absorbed through the vaginal walls (**Figure 6.3**). It is inserted into the vagina and removed after 3 weeks for 1 week and then a new one is inserted. The side effects are similar to other

Good practice point

Using the quick start method is simpler and more convenient and may reduce pregnancies while awaiting the correct 'time' to start the COCP.

Good practice point

The COCP should not be used in women taking some anti-epileptic drugs, as they accelerate metabolism of the hormones and increase failure rates. Women with epilepsy require careful pregnancy planning due to risks of seizure as well as teratogenicity of anti-epileptic medications. Other forms of contraception (e.g. Mirena) are more suitable in this population.

Clinical insight

Adequate COCP counselling is mandatory prior to prescribing this medication, as its efficacy depends directly on compliance and an understanding of how it works.

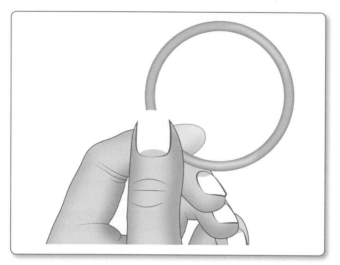

Figure 6.3 Vaginal ring (NuvaRing).

oestrogen-containing contraceptives including the COCP. Vaginal rings are more expensive than COCPs, but do not need to be taken every day.

Progesterone-only pill

The progesterone-only pill (POP) ('Minipill') works by thickening cervical mucus. It can also sometimes prevent ovulation. It comes in packets of 28 active pills (no 'sugar' pills). One pill is taken every day. Like the COCP, it needs to be taken at the same time every day; however, a pill is considered 'missed' if it is >3 hours late. If a pill is missed, alternative contraception (e.g. condoms) or abstinence is required for 3 days, while continuing to take the POP before protection against pregnancy is afforded.

The POP is a good option for women who are breastfeeding, as it does not interfere with the production of breast milk. It is also chosen by older women with contraindications for the COCP, if they decline long active reversible contraception due to low natural fertility. POP are associated with a higher rate of irregular breakthrough bleeding than COCP and provide lower contraceptive potency than COCP. This is why they are not used routinely in most women. There are newer high dose progestogen only pills containing drospirenone which have a similar missed dose window to COCP with stable bleeding patterns and these may be preferred by women who cannot take COCP but do not want a LARC.

Long-acting reversible

This category of contraceptives includes those that adopt a more 'set and forget' approach and are also reversible. These include depot medroxyprogesterone acetate (Depo-Provera), the progesterone implant (e.g. Implanon) and intra-uterine devices (IUDs) (e.g. Mirena). They are increasingly becoming recommended as first-line choices due to low failure rates (**Table 6.2**).

Depot medroxyprogesterone acetate

This is a progesterone-only injection that is administered intra-muscularly every 12 weeks by a healthcare professional. It works by preventing ovulation and thickening cervical mucus. It completely stops menses or makes bleeding much lighter, in the majority of women, although this takes time to develop (50% amenorrhoea at 12 months).

Progesterone implant

This is a 4 cm long and 3 mm thick flexible silicon rod, which is introduced sub-dermally using a needle introducer and local anaesthetic (**Figure 6.4**). It works by inhibiting ovulation and thickening cervical mucus. It lasts for up to 3 years when it can either be removed and replaced or removed altogether. Fertility returns quickly after removal.

Levonorgestrel intra-uterine device (e.g. Mirena intra-uterine device)

This is a small device, which is inserted transvaginally through the cervix into the uterine cavity (**Figure 6.5**). It contains a progesterone, levonorgestrel. It works by thickening cervical mucus and thins the lining of the uterus. It can be inserted

Method	Pearl index Typical (T) Perfect (P)	Advantages	Disadvantages and side effects	Non-contraceptive benefits
Depot medroxyprogesterone acetate	3 (T) 0.3 (P)	• Every 3 months • No oestrogen side effects • Does not interact with other medications	• Must be administered by health professional • Reversible decrease in bone mineral density • Delay in return to fertility of up to 24 months upon cessation • Irregular bleeding and weight gain in 20% • Once injection is given, must wait 3 months for any effect to wear off	High rate of iatrogenic amenorrhoea
Progesterone implant (e.g. Implanon)	0.05 (T) 0.05 (P)	• Lasts up to 3 years • Relatively non-invasive to insert (local anaesthetic) • Can be used where oestrogen is contraindicated	• Requires professional insertion • Irregular bleeding (30%)	Improvement in painful periods and may cause amenorrhoea (30%)
Levonorgestrel intra-uterine device (IUD) (e.g. Mirena)	0.1 (T) 0.1 (P)	Lasts up to 5 years	• Must be inserted trans-cervically • May be difficult to insert in women with a narrow cervical canal (e.g. nulliparous)	Improvement in painful periods and may cause amenorrhoea (30%)
Copper IUD	0.8 (T) 0.6 (P)	• Lasts 5–10 years depending on type • Non-hormonal	Can cause heavier and more painful periods in some	

Table 6.2 Long-acting contraception

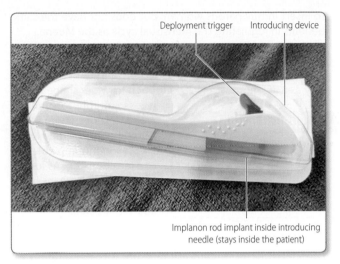

Deployment trigger   Introducing device

Implanon rod implant inside introducing
needle (stays inside the patient)

Figure 6.4 Implanon NXT.

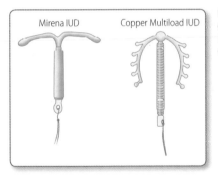

Mirena IUD   Copper Multiload IUD

Figures 6.5 Intra-uterine
devices (IUDs): (A) Mirena
IUD and (B) Multiload
copper IUD.

while awake in many women; although in nulliparous women,
it may not be easy to insert without cervical dilatation, in
which case, insertion under anaesthesia is recommended.
The Mirena IUD can be used to reduce menorrhagia and
dysmenorrhoea.

There is now also a smaller, lower dose levonorgestrel IUD
called a Kyleena. Because it is narrower, it is marginally easier

to insert in nulliparous women, but does not have the same benefits in regulating the menstrual cycle as the Mirena.

Copper intra-uterine device

This is a small device which is inserted into the uterus in the same way as a levonorgestrel IUD, although its wider shape makes it less suitable for nulliparous insertions (**Figure 6.5**). It is non-hormonal and works by preventing implantation of a fertilised egg. As for the levonorgestrel IUD, insertion can be more difficult in nulliparous women.

> **Clinical insight**
>
> If a woman is uncertain about whether or not she desires more children, a permanent form of contraception is not appropriate. This is especially as there are very effective long-acting reversible contraceptives also available.

Permanent

Permanent forms of contraception are excellent options for couples who have definitively completed their families. While some of these options can be mechanically 'reversed,' reversal does not equate to a return to normal fertility in many cases.

Tubal ligation

This is performed on the female partner usually laparoscopically or at the time of a caesarean section. A tubal ligation provides mechanical obstruction of the fallopian tubes, preventing the oocyte and sperm from meeting. It has no effect on hormones and for this reason, some women report heavier periods after ligation, as they stop using their usual oral contraceptive.

When done laparoscopically, Filshie clips are used to squeeze the tubes shut, with one placed on each tube, or the tubes are removed completely with a bipolar sealing device. At caesarean, due to tubal oedema that occurs during pregnancy, Filshie clips may not be sufficient and it is recommended that both tubes are cut, tied and diathermied (Pomeroy procedure) to prevent spontaneous re-anastomosis (**Figure 6.6**). Tubal ligation has a failure rate of approximately 1:250 at caesarean section. Laparoscopic tubal ligation has been largely replaced

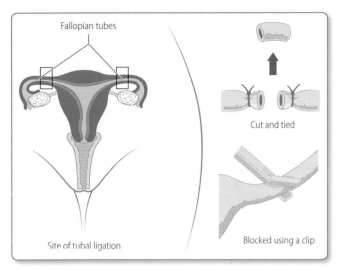

Figure 6.6 Tubal ligation with Filshie clips and tubal ligation with Pomeroy procedure.

by salpingectomies as this sterilises and provides risk reduction for future ovarian malignancy.

Vasectomy

This is performed on the male partner and can be done under local or general anaesthetic. Scrotal incisions are made and the vas deferens is identified and ligated bilaterally. This procedure is less risky to the male partner compared with a tubal ligation for the female partner, as entry into the peritoneal

Clinical insight

If a patient uses emergency contraception, a pregnancy test is performed 2 weeks afterwards to ensure that pregnancy has not occurred. This is because EC is not perfect and failure can occur; this chance increases with increasing time from unprotected intercourse to EC use.

Clinical insight

In a woman requesting emergency contraception, screen for STIs due to lack of barrier contraception. It is also important to enquire regarding sexual safety and offer support services.

cavity is not required. The failure rate for a vasectomy is approximately 1:2,000.

Emergency contraception

While not strictly a form of contraception, in women where contraception has not been used or contraception has failed (e.g. broken condom), emergency contraceptives (ECs) act to prevent ovulation and/or implantation.

High-dose progesterone pill

The most common form of EC is levonorgestrel 1.5 mg taken orally within 72 hours of intercourse. It is most effective when taken as soon as possible after intercourse, but has some effect up to 96 hours. It is the preferred agent, as it has the lowest incidence of unpleasant side effect such as nausea and vomiting and is safe in nearly all women. It has very few contraindications.

It is not as effective in women using drugs that induce liver enzymes such as rifampicin, phenytoin and carbamazepine. It is also not as effective in women with a body mass index (BMI) over 30 kg/m^2.

Pregnancy occurs in 2.2% overall, but this is higher with increasing interval from intercourse to use and is also higher in the follicular phase than luteal phase (as the woman is not at risk of unintended pregnancy if she is past her fertile window).

Ulipristal acetate

A 30-mg dose is taken orally within 120 hours of unprotected intercourse.

Concurrent use of progesterone contraceptives can reduce the efficacy of ulipristal acetate, so should not commence until 5 days after treatment.

Efficacy is reduced by liver enzyme-inducing

> ## Clinical insight
>
> In any woman being prescribed emergency contraception, long-term contraception should also be discussed and encouraged. It is important to know a Mirena is not effective as an EC and cannot be used for this indication.

medications as for levonorgestrel. Pregnancy occurs in 1.4% overall.

Copper intra-uterine device

This is the most effective form of emergency contraception with pregnancy occurring in <1%. It can be inserted up to 5 days after ovulation and can be left in situ for up to 5 years to provide ongoing contraception. It is, therefore, particularly useful in women who have regular cycles, are <5 days post-ovulation or have had multiple episodes of unprotected intercourse in the cycle. It is most useful in those who desire ongoing contraception.

6.4 Infertility

Most couples (85%) are able to achieve a pregnancy within 12 months of regular unprotected vaginal intercourse. A couple aged <35 years is considered to be 'infertile' if pregnancy has not been achieved within this time frame. While much of the history, examination and investigations centre around the female partner, male factor infertility accounts for approximately 40% of infertility.

Female factor

Female factor infertility refers to aetiologies of infertility that originate in the female. It includes central/ovulatory, tubal and uterine causes. Female factor aetiologies account for approximately 40% of infertility.

Central/Ovulatory

Central factors that can cause infertility in women include conditions that affect the hypothalamic-pituitary-gonadotropin axis. Women who are very underweight or elite athletes may experience

Clinical insight

When assessing a couple for infertility, it is essential not to forget the male partner.

Examination and investigation of the male partner are less invasive and lower risk when compared with equivalent examination and investigation of the female partner. Identification of a male factor might reduce the need for invasive testing of the female partner and significantly alter treatment course.

oligo-/anovulation. Other central factors include congenital abnormalities and disorders of sexual differentiation (see Chapter 3).

The most common cause of secondary ovulatory dysfunction is PCOS (see Chapter 4). This results in irregular menstrual cycles and infrequent or absent ovulation. Predicting the optimal time for intercourse to maximise fertility is difficult and the number of 'fertile days' per year is significantly reduced compared with a woman who cycles every 28 days.

Investigations A basal body temperature (taken before rising every morning with a sensitive thermometer) can be used to detect ovulation, as the average core body temperature rises by approximately 0.6°C after ovulation. A more useful marker of ovulation is serum mid-luteal progesterone. In irregular (or regular) cycles, the mid-luteal phase occurs 7 days before the expected next menses commences.

Urinary luteinising hormone (LH) prediction kits can also be used and are positive when LH excretion reaches a cut off level indicating the LH surge. For this to work, testing must occur daily starting from 3 days before the expected LH surge, as it is positive for only 1 day.

Karyotyping can be arranged in women where disorders of sexual differentiation are suspected. A good quality pelvic US scan will detect relevant Müllerian malformations and acquired uterine pathology such as sub-mucous fibroids or endometrial polyps.

Tubal

Tubal factor infertility is caused by tubal damage from infection, inflammation or surgery, which results in poorly functioning tubes. This is most commonly caused by pelvic inflammatory disease (see Chapter 5). Endometriosis and surgical adhesions as well as iatrogenic tubal damage (e.g. tubal ligation) are other common causes.

Clinical insight

Pelvic inflammatory disease increases the chance of ectopic pregnancy seven-fold and increases the chance of infertility with each episode.

Investigations There are two main methods of tubal assessment: (1) laparoscopic and (2) hysterosalpingogram.

During a hysterosalpingogram, a radiopaque dye is injected through the cervix and spillage is identified from the fimbrial ends of the tube using X-ray imaging. While this does not require an anaesthetic, it has a low positive predictive value but a high negative predictive value.

A laparoscopy with dye studies is optimal for identification of tubal occlusion, endometriosis and adhesive disease and has the advantage that if disease is identified, it can be treated simultaneously. In this procedure, the fimbrial ends of the tubes are visualised laparoscopically while instilling dye or saline through the cervix. Spillage is identified laparoscopically confirming tubal patency.

While these tests can confirm tubal patency, neither confirms tubal function.

Treatment In women with significant tubal damage, IVF is the ideal treatment for infertility.

In women with hydrosalpinges (where the fallopian tubes are blocked with fluid contents), salpingectomy with IVF is offered, as hydrosalpinges inhibit the success of IVF.

In women where tubal ligation is the cause of infertility, re-anastomosis is possible. Success is more likely if the woman is younger, rings or clips were used for ligation and there is no other cause of infertility. There is a 10% ectopic rate.

Uterine

Uterine causes of infertility are structural and include congenital malformations of which septate uterus is the most common cause of infertility (see Chapter 3). Fibroids, in particular submucous fibroids or large fibroids that result in cavity distortion (see Chapter 4), can also cause infertility. These may require surgical management prior to conception. Intra-uterine adhesions (Asherman syndrome), which are rare, but can be caused by repeated uterine surgery including hysteroscopic myomectomy, are also implicated. More commonly, endometrial polyps can cause infertility. These are usually easily removed hysteroscopically.

Investigations Hysterosalpingography is used to identify congenital abnormalities, fibroids, intra-uterine adhesions and polyps. These can also be identified with standard transvaginal ultrasound. The gold standard for diagnosis of uterine causes of infertility is hysteroscopy, as this allows simultaneous treatment and direct visualisation.

Male factor

Male factor infertility can be divided into pre-testicular, testicular and post-testicular causes (**Table 6.3**). Male factor infertility is almost exclusively treated with either donor sperm and intra-uterine insemination (IUI) or intra-cytoplasmic sperm injection (ICSI). The two main groups of problems are erectile and ejaculatory dysfunction and abnormalities of the sperm. Sperm abnormalities are divided into disorders of count ('oligospermia' = low and 'azoospermia' = nil), motility and shape (teratozoospermia).

Pre-testicular	• Klinefelter syndrome • Y chromosome micro-deletions • Hypothalamic/Pituitary tumour • Exogenous androgens/anabolic steroids • Idiopathic
Testicular	• Cryptorchidism • Varicocele • Mumps orchitis • Gonadotoxins (heat, smoking, heavy metals, solvents, marijuana and alcohol) • Other drugs (e.g. tetracyclines, spironolactone) • Anti-sperm antibodies • Prostatitis • Acrosomal failure
Post-testicular	• Vasectomy • Congenital bilateral absence of the vas deferens • Erectile dysfunction • Retrograde ejaculation

Table 6.3 Causes of male factor infertility

Investigations

A semen analysis is the basic mainstay of assessment of male factor infertility. It is taken after abstaining from ejaculation for 2–3 days, then ejaculating directly into a clean container (kept at body or room temperature) and examined within 1 hour. For accurate assessment, two samples should be taken 4 weeks apart.

Abnormal SA can resolve on repeat testing, as sperm production takes 60 days. Up to three SA are required to confirm an abnormality is genuine, as several environmental factors can temporarily impact semen quality.

Men with abnormal counts should have blood tests for follicle-stimulating hormone (FSH), LH, testosterone, prolactin and thyroid function to exclude medical causes.

To assess for structural testicular causes, a trans-rectal and trans scrotal ultrasound is performed to assess for obstruction and testicular masses, respectively. Genetic testing for cystic fibrosis (CF) mutation is performed to assess for atypical CF if obstructive azoospermia is identified (congenitally absent vas deferens). In men with severely abnormal semen analyses, karyotyping is performed for Klinefelter syndrome and Y chromosome micro deletions, as these both cause very low sperm counts.

Post-ejaculatory urine can be obtained with non-obstructive azoospermia to rule out retrograde ejaculation.

Treatment

Medical Hypogonadotropic hypogonadism [central deficiency in gonadotropin-releasing hormone (GnRH) and LH and FSH] can be treated with pulsatile GnRH, human chorionic gonadotropin (hCG), exogenous testosterone or pure FSH.

Retrograde ejaculation may benefit from sympathomimetics (e.g. imipramine, ephedrine and pseudo-ephedrine).

For any male factor infertility where at least some sperm are produced, ICSI is a valid option for fertility treatment. Otherwise, donor sperm is required.

Couple factor

A proportion (15–20%) of infertility has multiple minor contributors from both partners and this is referred to as 'couple factor.' A similar problem, unexplained infertility, occurs when all investigations for both the male and female partners are normal. In these couples, the treatment is usually IVF.

Assisted reproductive technologies

These are any medical techniques that can be used to treat infertility. They start with basic, minimally invasive methods and range up to IVF/ICSI.

Artificial insemination

This method of assisted reproduction is particularly useful in couples affected by ejaculatory dysfunction as long as the male can ejaculate for specimen collection. A sample of prepared (to remove prostaglandin as this causes painful uterine contractions) semen is injected through the cervix directly into the uterus just prior to ovulation. This is an effective and low-cost option in women without tubal factor or ovulatory dysfunction. It can also be used in combination with ovulation induction and has a small increase in pregnancy rate over natural intercourse (1–2%).

Donor sperm

In women without a male partner, azoospermia or where severe male factor exists, but the couple do not wish to use IVF, cryopreserved donor sperm can be used. Donor sperm is screened for infections and tested thoroughly prior to use. It can be used in any of the below forms of assisted reproductive technology (ART).

Ovulation induction

This process involves the use of a medication (such as clomiphene citrate or letrozole) designed to stimulate follicular development and ovulation and then timing intercourse around ovulation. This is mostly utilised for women with ovulatory dysfunction (e.g. PCOS) and works poorly with central causes of anovulation (prolactinoma, low BMI and stress). It works by decreasing oestrogen or blocking brain oestrogen receptors, causing release of more FSH from the pituitary gland.

Tablets are taken for 5 days early in the menstrual cycle and ovulation occurs around cycle day 14–19. 80% of women respond and half become pregnant over six cycles. There is a risk of multiple pregnancy (5–10% with Clomid).

Controlled ovarian hyperstimulation

This is the process where FSH injections are used to stimulate the development of a larger than usual number of ovarian follicles and oocytes. This is to maximise the yield of oocytes for IVF. Controlled ovarian hyperstimulation (COH) is also done for ovulation induction or insemination, but medication dose is much lower and only one to two mature follicles are created.

There are two phases to a traditional COH cycle: (1) down-regulation and (2) ovarian stimulation. Downregulation prevents breakthrough ovulation early in response to very high oestrogen levels later in the cycle. Stimulation recruits a supra-physiological pool of oocytes for retrieval. Other cycle protocols exist.

Ovarian suppression is achieved first with the contraceptive pill and GnRH agonist for 10 days, the pill is ceased, the agonist continues and gonadotropins are commenced to stimulate the ovaries. The aim is to recruit as many follicles as safely possible.

Intra-uterine insemination

This involves the introduction of washed, concentrated sperm via a catheter directly into the uterus just prior to expected ovulation. This can be used in combination with COH, but the regimen is different, as the aim is not to recruit too many oocytes.

This can be used to bypass male factor infertility (in particular ejaculatory dysfunction), but is not as effective as ICSI, which should be recommended after three failed cycles of IUI. It is also a good option in women without a partner or in a same-sex relationship.

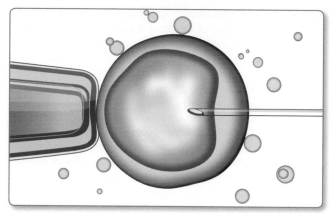

Figure 6.7 Intra-cytoplasmic sperm injection (ICSI).

In vitro fertilisation

This is a process where oocytes are retrieved after COH, fertilised with sperm outside the body in a petri dish, and the resulting embryo is inserted via a transcervical catheter into the endometrial cavity. This is the form of ART which is commonly used in women where less 'invasive' methods have not been successful and sperm function is normal.

Intra-cytoplasmic sperm injection

This is a type of IVF, but differs in that the sperm is injected directly into the oocyte (which has had all granulosa cells stripped from it) (**Figure 6.7**). This bypasses all steps in the natural conception process from ejaculation to the acrosomal reaction.

It is indicated in severe male factor, particularly severe oligoasthenospermia and in couples who have failed conventional IVF.

Steps in a typical IVF/ICSI cycle (note that different regimens exist):
• Controlled ovarian hyperstimulation using gonadotropins, oestradiol levels and transvaginal ultrasound to monitor follicular growth

- Prevention of premature LH surge and ovulation
- Oocyte maturation using trigger to simulate LH surge
- Oocyte retrieval
- Fertilisation by IVF/ICSI
- In vitro embryo culture
- Luteal support using vaginal progesterone
- Transfer of fresh embryos into the uterus and cryopreservation of excess embryos
- First trimester pregnancy monitoring

Complications of assisted reproductive technology

There are a number of complications that can result from ART. These include multiple gestation (e.g. twins or triplets), ovarian hyperstimulation syndrome (OHSS), ectopic and heterotopic pregnancy and depression and anxiety related to the stress of undergoing ART.

Ovarian hyperstimulation syndrome This is a serious condition that occurs when ovaries are over-stimulated. The exact pathophysiology is uncertain and can range from mild-to-severe disease.

Mild disease includes symptoms of nausea, abdominal pain and distension and enlarged ovaries of 5–12 cm in diameter. Moderate disease also presents with abdominal ascites. In its severest form, OHSS presents with clinically tense ascites, pleural effusions with shortness of breath, haemoconcentration, hypercoagulability, renal failure, pulmonary embolus and acute respiratory distress syndrome.

The management of OHSS is supportive until clinical condition improves spontaneously. This occurs quickly, if no embryo transfer has occurred, but can take many weeks to months to resolve if the woman is pregnant, as the hCG stimulates the ovaries further. It involves monitoring for complications of severe OHSS. This includes daily weight and

Clinical insight

Ovarian hyperstimulation syndrome can be life-threatening. It is important that women with OHSS are managed by a specialty unit and they are closely monitored for complications of OHSS. VTE is a cause of maternal death with OHSS and prophylaxis is essential.

girth, blood tests [full blood examination (FBE), urea elec-trolytes and creatinine (UEC), liver function test (LFT) and coagulation studies], thromboprophylaxis, slow intra-venous (IV) fluid maintenance and may require concentrated albumin infusions and paracentesis if effusions become severe and symptomatic.

6.5 First trimester bleeding

This is any vaginal bleeding that occurs in the first trimester of pregnancy. It can be very distressing, but the majority of women go onto have normal term deliveries. When a woman presents with first trimester bleeding, there are four possible pregnancy-related causes: (1) pregnancy of uncertain location, (2) miscarriage, (3) ectopic pregnancy and, rarely, (4) gestational trophoblastic disease (GTD).

The β-hCG in a normal pregnancy doubles every 48–72 hours in the early first trimester. This rate slows considerably after this point, plateaus at 10–12 weeks and then falls as the developing placenta takes over progesterone synthesis from the corpus luteum.

A falling β-hCG in the early first trimester is never normal and similarly slow-rising, or plateauing, β-hCG suggests ectopic or non-viable pregnancy. Be aware that management is rarely based on β-hCG alone, as this picture can be confused by different laboratory methods (15–20% difference in levels obtained in different labo-ratories), early twin demise and many other events. An ultrasound is more impor-tant once a gestational sac is identified.

When a woman presents with bleeding in early preg-nancy, the first priority is to determine haemodynamic stability. In a patient who

Clinical insight

In any woman with first trimester bleeding, it is important to exclude other sources of bleeding including bleeding originating from the cervix or vagina, rectum or bladder. This may be ascertained simply by taking a thorough history and examining appropriately.

Clinical insight

First trimester bleeding occurs in 30–40% of normal pregnancies, which go onto have a healthy baby at term.

presents unwell with features of haemoperitoneum or exsanguination (tachycardia, hypotension and/or 'acute' abdomen), it is imperative that resuscitation occurs simultaneously to assessment. Large-bore IV access with FBE, cross-match and serum β hCG are ordered. High-flow oxygen is applied via Hudson mask. IV crystalloid is commenced immediately while waiting for blood to arrive.

> ## Clinical insight
>
> After 10–12 weeks, the beta-human chorionic gonadotropin (β-hCG) in a normal pregnancy will start to decline. This occurs as the placenta takes over 'management' of the pregnancy. Therefore, it is of no concern when the β-hCG falls after 12 weeks, as long as a fetal heart beat is still present. This also means that after a fetus is seen on ultrasound, there is no indication for β-hCG to confirm viability.

Once haemodynamic stability has been confirmed (or instability has been corrected), two factors need to be determined – where the pregnancy is *located* and whether or not it is *viable* (alive). In order to assess this, a transvaginal ultrasound is required.

Pregnancy of unknown location

This is a condition when a woman presents with a positive β-hCG and a transvaginal ultrasound showing an 'empty' uterus. Management of this clinical presentation depends largely on the haemodynamic stability of the woman.

If she is *unstable* with an acute abdomen, immediate laparoscopy (with or without laparotomy) is indicated for presumed ruptured ectopic pregnancy.

If there is no acute abdomen, but the woman is bleeding from her uterus, an urgent pelvic ultrasound

> ## Clinical insight
>
> With a serum β-hCG level of >1,500 IU/L, one would expect to locate a pregnancy in the uterus on vaginal scan. If a gestational sac cannot be seen at this level of β-hCG, this is usually either a complete miscarriage or an ectopic pregnancy.

> ## Clinical insight
>
> 'Pregnancy of unknown location' is not a diagnosis, but rather an indication that further testing is required before a diagnosis can be reached.

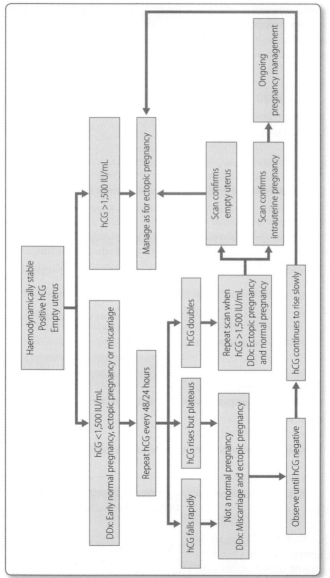

Figure 6.8 Assessing a pregnancy of unknown location. (DDx, differential diagnosis; hCG, human chorionic gonadotropin)

Type	Clinical findings	Diagnosis
Missed miscarriage	• Loss of pregnancy symptoms • Minimal or no bleeding • No passage of products of conception	A routine ultrasound for dating or viability assessment detects a fetus without a fetal heart beat or two ultrasounds done 1–2 weeks apart show inadequate growth in the gestational sac or embryo
Incomplete miscarriage	• Ongoing vaginal bleeding • Passage of products of conception • Loss of pregnancy symptoms	An ultrasound will show heterogeneous and sometimes vascular material within the uterus and no fetal heartbeat. The beta-human chorionic gonadotropin (β-hCG) will drop
Complete miscarriage	Vaginal bleeding and passage of products of conception and then resolution of all symptoms including bleeding	An ultrasound will show an empty uterus. The β-hCG will drop rapidly
Threatened miscarriage	Vaginal bleeding with no passage of products of conception. Pregnancy symptoms may or may not continue	An ultrasound performed after the bleeding shows a fetus with a heartbeat
Septic miscarriage	Fever, rigors and signs of sepsis. Purulent vaginal discharge and vaginal bleeding	An ultrasound shows the absence of a fetal heartbeat. There are clinical features of uterine infection and sepsis

Table 6.4A Types of miscarriage

is indicated. These steps are taken while concurrently resuscitating the woman as discussed above.

If the woman is haemodynamically *stable*, time can be taken to determine an exact diagnosis before choosing the appropriate course of management. This usually involves a repeat β-hCG every 48 hours until either the β-hCG rises to above 1,500 IU/L, when an ultrasound can be performed or

Type of miscarriage	Pregnancy symptoms	Vaginal bleeding	Products of conception passed	Signs of infection	Fetal heartbeat seen on ultrasound	β-hCG trend
Missed	−	−	−	−	−	→
Incomplete	±	+	+	−	−	→
Complete	−	+	+	−	−	→
Threatened	+	+	−	−	+	←
Septic	−	+	±	+	−	→

Table 6.4B Types of miscarriage

the β-hCG falls (**Figure 6.8**). Once the diagnosis is made, management can proceed depending on the location of the pregnancy and its viability (Page 165).

Clinical insight

Miscarriage does not always present with bleeding and bleeding does not always represent a miscarriage.

Clinical insight

The term 'abortion' should no longer be used due to stigma. Miscarriages are termed as 'miscarriage' or 'pregnancy loss.' 'Termination' is used to describe what was previously described as an 'abortion.'

Miscarriage

First trimester miscarriage is diagnosed in the absence of a fetal heart beat with a fetus of ≥7 mm in length on vaginal scan or a failure for the embryo to grow appro-priately over a 1–2 week period in an intra-uterine pregnancy. There are several types of miscarriage (**Table 6.4**). Miscarriage management is based on ultrasound findings rather than clinical findings alone.

Diagnosis

Some women experience sudden loss of pregnancy symptoms (such as nausea and vomiting), vaginal bleeding or lower abdominal cramps, but many women have no symptoms. Therefore, an accurate diagnosis of miscarriage is impossible to make based on history or examination alone.

Diagnosis relies on two investigations: (1) a quantitative serum β-hCG and (2) transvaginal ultrasound. Even with these, if performed very early in pregnancy, a definitive diagnosis may not be able to be made from one test alone and serial investigations may be required.

A falling β-hCG in the early first trimester signals a non-viable pregnancy. This may either be an ectopic pregnancy or a miscarriage. Once a transvaginal ultrasound identifies an intra-uterine gestation, ultrasound (rather than serial β-hCG) should then be used to monitor its growth. If a transvaginal ultrasound performed 1–2 weeks after the first still fails to show a fetal heartbeat when the fetus is ≥7 mm in length or the gestational sac remains empty and ≥25 mm in size or there is no heartbeat and inadequate growth of the fetus, missed miscarriage is confirmed.

Management

The first step in management is to determine maternal haemodynamic stability. If the woman is well and bleeding is not affecting her haemodynamic status, three options are available for management: (1) expectant, (2) medical and (3) surgical. Either option is appropriate.

Expectant management involves serial β-hCG every 1–2 weeks until the β-hCG becomes negative. For an incomplete miscarriage, this is successful in approximately 60% of cases. In a missed miscarriage, success is closer to 40%.

Medical management involves using the prostaglandin misoprostol to soften and open the cervix and cause uterine contractions to expel the products of conception. This is effective in 60% of missed miscarriage and up to 90% of incomplete miscarriages.

Both expectant management and medical management should only be allowed 1–2 weeks to work. In this time, there is no increased risk of infection. Failing this, surgical management is required.

Surgical management involves a general anaesthetic and suction curettage, where a narrow tube is inserted into the cervix with theatre wall suction applied to evacuate the contents of the uterus. This is commonly performed without ultrasound guidance and is 95% successful at emptying the uterus in its entirety.

In a haemodynamically unstable woman, resuscitation occurs and a suction curettage must be performed as soon as possible as this will stop the bleeding.

Ectopic pregnancy

An ectopic pregnancy is a pregnancy that develops outside the uterus. They most commonly develop in the fallopian tubes, but can also develop in the ovaries, cervix, caesarean scars and abdominal cavity. The baseline risk of ectopic pregnancy is 1.6% and the risk of recurrence after one ectopic pregnancy is up to 10%. A ruptured ectopic pregnancy is a gynaecological emergency and requires urgent surgical management. However, an ectopic that has not ruptured can be managed with medical treatment. The following discussion covers tubal ectopic pregnancies. Ectopics in other locations require specialist management.

Diagnosis

When taking a history regarding possible ectopic pregnancy, in addition to a standard medical history, screen for risk factors including tubal surgery/damage, endometriosis/adhesions/appendicitis, pelvic inflammatory disease, smoking and failed progesterone contraception (including emergency contraception and Mirena IUD). Enquire regarding peritonitic and shoulder tip pain and symptoms of blood loss (fainting, nausea and vomiting) as these suggest ectopic rupture.

On examination, there may or may not be adnexal tenderness or signs of an acute abdomen (e.g. rigidity, cross-tenderness, rebound tenderness). Vaginal bleeding is not always a presenting feature.

Arrange blood tests for β-hCG (confirm pregnancy!) or at least urine hCG in an emergency (can be a catheter specimen), blood group and screen (potential surgery, need for anti-D, if Rh negative), and transvaginal ultrasound, if stable.

Once an ultrasound identifies an ectopic pregnancy, management can proceed. Unstable women are diagnosed at emergency surgery.

Management

Management options depend on clinical stability and the risk of ectopic rupture.

Expectant management is an option for women with hCG <1,000 IU/L and declining with no clinical symptoms of rupture (abdominal pain or haemodynamic instability). If this is employed, it is essential that the patient be aware to return to hospital immediately should she develop abdominal pain. In addition, she requires serial hCG monitoring until the hCG is negative.

Medical management can be offered in tubal ectopics with a low risk of rupture. These women must have minimal pain, minimal free pelvic fluid (blood), a β-hCG <5,000 IU/L, no fetal heart beat, a gestational sac <4 cm in diameter and be willing and able to attend for regular serial β-hCG and follow-up.

Medical management is with methotrexate 1 mg/kg intramuscular (IM) in a single dose for tubal ectopics.

Clinical insight

An ectopic pregnancy can rupture at *any* positive level of hCG, even if it is low.

Clinical insight

When methotrexate is given to manage ectopic pregnancy, there is often an increase in β-hCG from day 1 to day 3. This is not of concern as long as the patient remains asymptomatic and the hCG subsequently drops.

Serial β-hCG is required on day 1 (day of administration), day 4 and day 7 and then up to every week until negative. If treatment is likely to be successful, there will be a drop in hCG from day 4 to day 7 of at least 15%. Pregnancy is contra-indicated for 3 months after treatment as methotrexate is teratogenic.

An unstable patient at any positive level of β-hCG requires urgent resuscitation. Attention is paid to response, airway management, circulation and restoring blood volume immediately. Following stabilisation, surgical management is undertaken.

Surgical management, with laparoscopic salpingectomy, is used in women who have signs of a ruptured ectopic or when any of the criteria for medical management (above) are not satisfied or if the woman requests it. Occasionally, a laparotomy is required, but this is unusual and reserved for cases where rapid and safe laparoscopic entry cannot be achieved in major intra-abdominal haemorrhage.

A salpingostomy (incising the tube and extruding the ectopic) is also uncommonly performed, as this result in further tubal damage and does not improve outcomes. It may be considered in women with only one uterine tube who do not wish to use IVF in future.

Gestational trophoblastic disease

This encompasses a number of conditions where abnormal gestational trophoblastic tissue proliferates within the uterus and can metastasise. It occurs when there is an error during fertilisation and two sperm fertilise one ovum or an empty ovum is fertilised by two sperm, as these all lead to unbalanced ratio of maternal to paternal genetics. The most common forms of GTD are complete molar pregnancy and partial molar pregnancy. These can only be accurately differentiated on histology (**Table 6.5**) and can progress to choriocarcinoma. Placental site trophoblastic tumour is another rare form of GTD that requires hysterectomy.

Molar pregnancies are characterised by a very high β-hCG concentration.

> ## Clinical insight
>
> The risk of recurrence of a molar pregnancy is 1:80 after one mole and 20% after two moles.
>
> Making an accurate diagnosis of the type of molar pregnancy requires karyotyping; this is important because the risk of developing gestational neoplasia and recurrence risk is higher for complete molar pregnancy than partial molar pregnancy.
>
> Karyotyping cannot be performed on tissue stored in formalin.

Feature	Partial molar pregnancy	Complete molar pregnancy
Fetal/Embryonic tissue	Present	Absent
Hydatidiform swelling of chorionic villi	Focal	Diffuse
Trophoblastic hyperplasia	Focal	Diffuse
Scalloping of chorionic villi	Present	Absent
Trophoblastic stromal inclusions	Present	Absent
Karyotype	Triploid 69,XXY	46,XX and 46,XY

Table 6.5 Comparison of complete and partial molar pregnancy

Partial molar pregnancy

This occurs when an oocyte is fertilised by two sperm. It commonly results in a triploid 69,XXY karyotype. This rarely progresses to metastatic choriocarcinoma. A pelvic US may show fetal parts and a heartbeat.

Complete molar pregnancy

This occurs when an enucleated oocyte is fertilised by two sperm or fertilised by one sperm which then duplicates its deoxyribonucleic acid (DNA). This has a risk of progression to malignancy of 4%. Ultrasound shows a characteristic 'snow-storm' appearance or a vesicular 'bunch of grapes' appearance from aberrant placental development. Patients may present with vaginal bleeding, a uterus that is larger than dates, hyper-emesis, hypertension or pre-eclampsia, hyperthyroidism and large ovarian theca lutein cysts in low-resource settings. Most women in industrialised nations are diagnosed on first trimester US scan either for bleeding or for routine pregnancy dating.

Management

Once the woman is stabilised from a vaginal bleeding point of view, an urgent suction curettage is performed, with the products of conception kept in saline and sent for karyotyping and histopathology. Anti-D is administered, if appropriate.

Weekly β-hCGs are performed until negative for 3 weeks and then monthly until the hCG is negative for at least 6 months. During this time, the woman is asked to use effective contraception, as a rise in hCG from a new pregnancy will be difficult to differentiate from a recurrence of disease.

6.6 Recurrent pregnancy loss

Recurrent pregnancy loss (RPL) is defined as three consecutive miscarriages before 20 weeks of gestation. It affects 1% of couples.

Pathophysiology

The main risk factors for RPL are maternal age and previous miscarriages. As a woman gets older, the likelihood of chromosomal errors within the oocyte climbs and these chromosomal errors cause early death of the developing embryo. Paternal age also has an impact on RPL, albeit lesser. The risk of a subsequent miscarriage climbs after each miscarriage, reaching 40% after three consecutive losses.

Obesity, smoking and alcohol consumption also increase the risk of RPL. These modifiable factors should be corrected where possible.

Anti-phospholipid syndrome is the major known treatable cause of RPL.

Inherited chromosomal abnormalities also can result in RPL. If either parent carries a translocation (commonly a reciprocal or Robertsonian translocation) or if both parents carry the same genetic abnormality, this can result in RPL. This affects 1–2% of RPL couples.

Some congenital uterine malformations, cervical weakness, thyroid dysfunction and poorly controlled diabetes and thrombophilias have all been implicated in RPL.

Clinical insight

Anti-phospholipid syndrome requires a combination of clinical criteria and biochemical criteria.

Clinical criteria:

- At least one clinical event including an arterial, venous or small vessel thrombus
- *A specific pregnancy complication:*
  o ≥One loss of a normal fetus ≥10 weeks of gestation
  o ≥Three consecutive spontaneous losses <10 weeks of gestation
  o ≥One birth of a morphologically normal neonate <34 weeks of gestation due to eclampsia or severe pre-eclampsia or severe growth restriction

Biochemical criteria:

- An elevated anti-cardiolipin, anti-beta-2-glycoprotein I or lupus anticoagulant detected on two occasions separated by 12 weeks

Clinical insight

Pre-implantation genetic screening involves taking a cell biopsy from an in vitro embryo and analysing karyotype. Only embryos with a normal karyotype are transferred to the uterus. It is useful to prevent introduction of a chromosomally abnormal embryo into the uterus. It requires IVF.

Investigations

These are based on potential treatable causes.

Anti-phospholipid antibodies, cytogenetic analysis of products of conception on the third miscarriage, karyotyping of the woman and her partner, pelvic ultrasound and a thrombophilia screen (for second trimester losses) are performed. Testing for thyroid function and diabetes is also completed.

Management

Treatment is directed at any identified cause.

Anti-phospholipid syndrome is treated with low-dose aspirin and prophylactic low-molecular-weight heparin.

If an abnormal parental karyotype is identified, referral to a clinical geneticist is necessary and consideration for IVF with pre-implantation genetic screening is appropriate.

Congenital uterine anomalies can be treated surgically, but this does not appear to prevent further miscarriage and is now not recommended for this reason.

Cervical weakness can be treated with cervical surveillance and/or cervical cerclage or progesterone depending on the clinical situation.

It is uncertain whether progesterone and β-hCG supplementation prevent RPL. Progesterone has some evidence base where bleeding exists and is also very safe and, therefore, often utilised.

In women with thrombophilias, low-molecular-weight heparin can be used in those with recurrent second trimester loss, but does not prevent first trimester loss.

The psychological impact of RPL cannot be under-estimated and multi-disciplinary care involving a psychologist and/or a psychiatrist is essential. The couple is reassured that if no cause is found, there is a reasonable chance (>70%) of successful pregnancy next time.

6.7 Termination of pregnancy

Termination of pregnancy (previously known as 'abortion') involves the intentional cessation of a currently viable pregnancy. Indications and legality of termination vary considerably across countries and even within the same country. The two main groups of termination are social and medical. Medical termination is permissible in many settings, but social termination is globally more tightly restricted.

The ethics of termination is beyond the scope of this book; however, it should be noted that the woman's choice and consent are imperative when making clinical decisions about the progress of her pregnancy.

Pathophysiology

Pathological reasons for interrupting a pregnancy include maternal severe disease and fetal severe disease.

Maternal severe disease includes conditions where the mother requires the pregnancy to be terminated to allow lifesaving treatment such as cancer chemotherapy or where continuing the pregnancy has an unacceptable risk of maternal death such as in Eisenmenger's syndrome and pulmonary hypertension where the chance of death is up to 50%.

Fetal indications include major non-survivable or life-altering structural abnormalities, such as trisomy, anencephaly or major cardiac defects and in situationswhere survival to a viable healthy birth is very unlikely, such as in pre-viable rupture of the membranes or pre-viable severe pre-eclampsia.

Counselling

The woman's reasons for requesting termination (medical, fetal and social) are discussed and options for alternate care are discussed, if this has not previously been done. She is counselled about the psychological impact of termination and what to expect before, during and after the termination. She is also counselled about post-termination contraception, especially in cases where the termination occurred due to an unwanted pregnancy ('social' termination).

After 20 weeks, she is also advised about options for lactation suppression (e.g. with cabergoline).

In women having a termination for fetal anomalies, a post-mortem evaluation of the fetus is also offered. Anti-D is administered in non-isoimmunised rhesus-negative women.

Management

Available methods for termination depend on the gestation at termination, woman's wishes and prior uterine surgery.

Terminations occurring <14 weeks can be performed surgically with a suction curettage or medically with mifepristone/misoprostol. Beyond this gestation, terminations are ideally performed with a medical induction of labour.

In terminations occurring at close-to-viable gestations (>22 weeks of gestation), the trans-uterine injection of fetal intra-cardiac potassium chloride, prior to induction, is offered to prevent a live baby being born.

Surgical termination

This involves a general anaesthetic and a suction curettage, often under ultrasound guidance at later gestations >12 weeks to ensure complete evacuation and to avoid uterine perforation.

Pre-operative misoprostol administration 2–4 hours before the procedure facilitates dilatation and should be offered.

Medical termination

At early gestations <9 weeks, this is performed with mifepristone and misoprostol given sequentially. This regimen also works at later gestations, but requires admission to hospital as pain, bleeding and complication rates such as retained placenta are common. Some settings use misoprostol alone for legal or financial reasons, but this is associated with longer duration and lower success rates.

For third trimester terminations, which are uncommon, low-dose misoprostol or a routine induction of labour with oxytocin can be used. Mifepristone can also be used. Medical terminations often take 24–48 hours to complete. These medications are not available for this indication in all countries.

Following termination, referral to a social worker and grievance counsellor is considered, depending on the case.

6.8 Violence against women and informed consent

Violence against women is defined by the United Nations as any act of gender-based violence that results in, or is likely to result in, physical, sexual, or mental harm or suffering to women, including threats of such acts, coercion or arbitrary deprivation of liberty, whether occurring in public or in private life.

It is common with almost 30% of all women who have been in any relationship having experienced some form of violence.

Because of the prevalence, it is essential to consider violence against women in every presentation that they review.

> **Clinical insight**
>
> Contrary to popular belief, the perpetrator of violence is most often known to the woman and is commonly their partner. Attacks by strangers are much less common.

Each claim of violence must be approached sensitively and taken seriously. At the request of the woman, it should be referred to the appropriate local authorities. It is important to remember that unless the woman gives consent, a healthcare professional cannot break her confidentiality and report to the authorities (except if she is a child or a child is at risk). This may vary by jurisdiction.

Menopause

7.1 Introduction

Menopause is a normal and universal experience for all women who reach the age of 51 (on average). Menopause occurs as the oocyte pool is exhausted, resulting in a cessation of ovarian sex steroid production and a permanent transition to very low serum oestrogen levels.

Most symptoms of menopause directly relate to low oestrogen and can cause considerable bother. As half of the population experiences menopause, it is important to be aware of the physiology, symptoms and treatment options for menopause and be able to provide appropriate reassurance and advice.

Clinical insight

In most women, menopause is a clinical diagnosis and occurs when a woman has not had a period for >12 months. A blood test for elevated follicle-stimulating hormone (FSH) is not required for diagnosis; however, it may be useful in women who have had a hysterectomy or in very young women where premature ovarian insufficiency is suspected.

7.2 Clinical scenario

A 50-year-old para 2 attends for review due to bothersome nocturnal sweating, she is changing soaked sheets several times every night and has poor sleep as a result. She is exhausted and teary during the consultation. She also reports low libido and dyspareunia and relationship difficulties with several recent fights with her partner. She experiences hot flushes many times each day.

Apart from asthma and well-controlled hypertension on irbesartan, there is no other history of note and body mass index (BMI) is normal. She has previously had a tubal ligation. She does not smoke.

She attends seeking an explanation for her symptoms and treatment and directly enquires regarding 'herbal pills' sold in the chemist.

Further history taking reveals that her menstrual cycle has been increasingly erratic for 12 months with her last menstrual period occurring 3 months ago and remission of her symptoms when her cycle returns. She denies symptoms of associated headache, severe hypertension, infection, heat or cold intolerance, weight change or other systemic concern.

Her mother's menopause occurred at the age of 50 years and there is no personal or family history of breast, ovarian or endometrial cancer or venous thromboembolism (VTE).

Examination shows a tired appearing middle-aged woman. Blood pressure is 130/75 mmHg. Thyroid, abdominal and cardiovascular examination is unremarkable. Genital examination also shows pale vaginal and vulval tissue with a dry appearance.

Diagnostic approach

This case is a classic presentation of peri-menopause with both systemic (sweats, flushes, sleep and mood) and genital symptoms related to low oestrogen. This is supported by her age, an absence of symptoms to support sepsis, thyroid disease, carcinoid syndrome or phaeochromocytoma. The irregularity of her periods with increasing duration of amenorrhoea between cycles and remission of symptoms when her periods do occur also support the diagnosis.

Clinical investigations

Serum levels of FSH and luteinising hormone (LH) vary significantly during peri-menopause. They are difficult to interpret for this reason and do not usually change management. They should only be performed where the diagnosis is uncertain, ideally on cycle day 3. Similarly, pelvic ultrasound is reserved for cases where endometrial hyperplasia is suspected due to heavy prolonged menses.

Management

The woman is provided with reassurance that her symptoms are caused by menopause, which is a physiological (therefore, normal) event, but as her symptoms are significantly affecting her quality of life, treatment is indicated and hormone replacement is both the most effective and safe option.

She is also informed her genital symptoms can be treated with topical oestrogen and this is also very safe.

Written information is given regarding menopause, non-hormonal and hormonal treatment options and the woman commences transdermal oestrogen with a levonorgestrel intrauterine system (Mirena) to also help control the nuisance aspect of irregular infrequent menses.

Her cervical screening test is updated as it is overdue, a request for screening mammogram and discussion of factors affecting bone density (exercise and vitamin D) and bowel screening is also performed.

She leaves with a plan for review in 3 months.

7.3 Physiology of menopause

As introduced in the beginning of this chapter, menopause is inevitable for all cycling women. This is because unlike the testes where spermatogenesis occurs throughout adult life, ovaries contain a finite pool of primordial follicles that are formed in embryonic development and decline steadily throughout childhood and reproductive life (**Figure 7.1**).

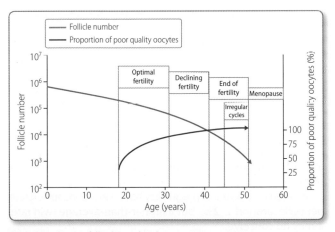

Figure 7.1 Ovarian follicular pool and menopause transition.

After menarche, growth of follicles in response to FSH causes normal oestradiol levels and ovulation/menstrual cycles.

Once only a few viable follicles exist to make oestradiol, FSH levels rise with ovulation and menstrual cycles become progressively more irregular with frequent anovulation culminating in cessation of ovulation (menopause).

Menopause is not an all-or-nothing event, can fluctuate, and the transition begins up to a decade earlier than permanent secondary amenorrhoea. It is divided into pre-menopausal, peri-menopausal, menopausal and finally post-menopausal phases (**Figure 7.2**).

Menopause that occurs before the age of 45 years is defined as early, but it is not necessarily pathological. This is more likely in smokers, those with a family history of early menopause and those who have had prior chemotherapy or ovarian surgery.

Menopause before the age of 40 years is defined as premature [premature menopause (PM), better termed as premature ovarian insufficiency (POI), as it is not always absolute and permanent], is more likely to be pathological and should be investigated further (see below).

Pre-menopausal phase

This phase starts in the early to mid-40s. Mild elevation of FSH is required to stimulate the ovaries, causing intermittent disordered ovulation with one, two or no oocytes recruited in variable amounts. The woman may report worsening menstrual headaches due to lower background oestrogen in early follicular phase and menorrhagia due to anovulatory bleeding. She may also experience intermittent high oestrogen concentrations resulting in disordered endometrial growth when several follicles are recruited. The fine balance of normal ovulatory mechanisms begins to become deranged. Cycles become irregular.

Vasomotor symptoms and atrophic symptoms do not occur as most of the time, oestrogen concentrations are still relatively normal.

Women who attempt pregnancy have a low conception rate per cycle (around 1–2%), but a higher-than-average twin rate, if they do conceive.

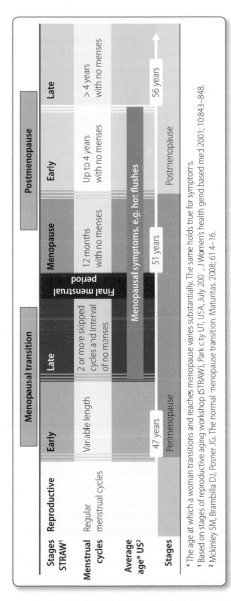

Stages STRAW[1]	Reproductive	Menopausal transition		Postmenopause		
		Early	Late	Menopause	Early	Late
Menstrual cycles	Regular menstrual cycles	Variable length	2 or more skipped cycles and interval of no menses	12 months with no menses	Up to 4 years with no menses	> 4 years with no menses
Average age* US[2]		47 years		51 years		56 years
Stages		Perimenopause			Postmenopause	

Final menstrual period

Menopausal symptoms, e.g. hot flushes

* The age at which a woman transitions and reaches menopause varies substantially. The same holds true for symptoms.

[1] Based on stages of reproductive aging workshop (STRAW), Park City UT, USA, July 2001; J Women's health gend based med 2001; 10:843–848.

[2] Mckinley SM, Brambilla DJ, Posner JG. The normal menopause transition. Maturitas. 2008; 61:4–16.

Figure 7.2 Menopause phases.

Peri-menopausal phase

This occurs when very few oocytes remain and predate cessation of menses by around 12 months. In this phase, follicular development and oestrogen production are variable and oestrogen deficiency symptoms occur. Menstrual cycles are infrequent and irregular and episodes of anovulatory heavy bleeding and metrostaxis can also occur.

Spontaneous pregnancy is rare.

Menopausal phase

In this phase, after the last menstrual period, oestrogen deficiency symptoms become prominent. Very low concentrations of oestrogen exist, the oocyte pool is permanently depleted and amenorrhoea occurs.

Post-menopausal phase

This phase is diagnosed in retrospect when 12 months of secondary amenorrhoea have occurred. Oestrogen deficiency symptoms generally improve, but may not cease. Many women continue to have bothersome vasomotor symptoms for up to a decade (and occasionally beyond) after menopause.

Contraception can be safely ceased at this time.

7.4 Clinical features and investigations

The clinical features of menopause relate to oestrogen deficiency, disordered ovulation and, as a result, disordered progesterone production. Healthy women with menopausal symptoms at the expected age (over 45 years) do not require investigation.

Clinical features can be divided into systemic and genital, as this neatly identifies the best treatment options for each. In general, systemic symptoms respond to systemic therapy, which can be given orally or transdermally, while local genitourinary symptoms are effectively treated with local topical therapy and do not require systemic treatment options.

Systemic and genital features are outlined below in **Tables 7.1** and **7.2**.

Systemic feature	Symptoms	Signs
Vasomotor symptom (VMS)	Sudden feeling of overheating, described as rising up from the feet to the head	• Behavioural response – removal of excess clothing, fanning self and cool cloths • Facial and chest erythema
	• Sweats at night – usually wake up with soaked sheets • Poor sleep, frequent night wakes and fatigue	If examined during an episode – wet skin/sweat. Rare to capture this
Ovulatory dysfunction	Recruitment of no follicle/low oestrogen – night sweats and VMS	• Usually no oestrogen deficiency signs, until no follicle recruitment becomes frequent • Thinning of skin, dryness and hair thinning and increased facial hair
	Anovulation – delay in menses and eventual anovulatory menorrhagia	Signs of iron deficiency anaemia
	Poly-follicular recruitment – ovulatory menorrhagia due to high oestrogen stimulation of endometrium	Irregular menstrual cycle length
Joint pain	Painful joints – generally poly-articular – due to effect of loss of oestrogen on pain pathways and chondrocytes	Normal joint on examination and no signs of synovitis
Formication	Sensation of crawling under skin surface – often distressing	Normal examination and no signs of peripheral neuropathy
Low mood and forgetfulness	Self-reported, multifactorial – poor sleep [central nervous system (CNS)] and oestrogen deficiency	No evidence of dementing process

Table 7.1 Systemic features of early menopause transition

Genitourinary feature	Symptoms	Signs
Atrophy	Superficial dyspareunia	Pallor of vulva/vagina
	Vulvo-vaginal dryness	Dry appearance
	Light bleeding	Petechial haemorrhage on speculum examination
Urinary	• Urinary frequency • Urinary urgency • New stress incontinence	• Negative urinalysis • Positive leak from urethra with coughing

Table 7.2 Genitourinary features of menopause

Clinical insight

Women who are never exposed to oestrogen do not suffer from menopausal symptoms, thus untreated primary amenorrhoea due to hypogonadism is not associated with vasomotor symptoms or night sweats.

Once the brain/hypothalamus is primed by exposure to physiological oestrogen, however, menopausal symptoms inevitably result, if this is removed.

The severity of symptoms varies between women; thin women tend to report more severe symptoms than obese women. This is because fat produces oestrone, which is less biologically potent than oestradiol (the normal pre-menopausal major circulating oestrogen), but is able to stimulate the oestrogen receptor. This also places obese women at increased risk of endometrial hyperplasia in the post-menopausal phase due to chronic oestrone stimulation of the endometrium in the absence of progesterone.

Surgical menopause also causes more severe and abrupt symptoms, as the entire gonadal sex steroid output is abruptly ceased.

Early menopause affects around 10% of women and POI occurs in 4%.

Women with suspected early menopause or POI should have confirmation with pelvic ultrasound (few follicles on ovaries and thin endometrial stripe) and serum FSH and LH levels on two separate occasions >6 weeks apart. If these are persistently elevated (>25 IU/L), early menopause or POI is diagnosed.

As POI has a higher chance of genetic, endocrine or immuno-logical pathological cause, investigate further with a karyotype and fragile X genetic test (as mosaic Turner syndrome and fragile X also cause POI). Also screen for associated autoimmune diseases (lupus, thyroid, antiadrenal and ovarian antibodies) and consider baseline assessment of cardiovascular and bone health/risk factors.

7.5 Sequelae

Sequelae of menopause are divided into early and late. Women experience these to varying degrees and women who have no, minimal or are not troubled by their symptoms do not require treatment if their menopause occurs after 45 years. Women who have an early (under 45 years) or premature (under 40 years) menopause require hormone replacement at least until the age of 50 years and can be reassessed at this time. This is because late sequelae will happen earlier in these groups with a greater lifespan to suffer the consequences of poor bone mineral density and other issues related to prolonged oestrogen deficiency.

Early sequelae include the symptoms outlined in **Table 7.1** above with the most important effects being mood distur-bance, poor well-being, function and sleep.

Late sequelae are the result of prolonged oestrogen defi-ciency on the cardiovascular, skeletal, integumentary and genital systems.

Cardiovascular

Oestrogen loss causes increased rates of atherosclerosis forma-tion and reduced nitric oxide-mediated vascular relaxation. This results in elevation in the rate of peripheral vascular disease, myocardial infarction and stroke in the post-menopausal population.

Early initiation of hormone replacement may be beneficial in reducing this risk, but late initiation is not probably because much of the macrovascular 'damage is done.'

Skeletal

Oestrogen loss results in reduced osteoblastic activity and increased osteoclastic activity. Bone mass inevitably declines continuously for many years and if menopause is early, lifespan is very long or peak bone mass in young adulthood is suboptimal, osteoporosis (T-score <2.5 standard deviations from standard young adult) will occur and with it the risk of fractures (**Figure 7.3**).

Integument and connective tissue

Collagen levels decline and the skin thins, becomes more wrinkled and drier in many women.

Loss of oestrogen also reduces inhibition on male pattern hair changes. Thinning of scalp hair (female pattern baldness) and development of chin hair can occur – this is often particularly distressing.

Loss of strength also occurs more generally in connective tissue and this contributes to pelvic organ prolapse.

Genitourinary tract

The bladder trigone, urethra, vulval and vaginal mucosa contain oestrogen receptors and these tissues undergo atrophic

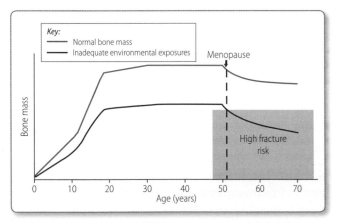

Figure 7.3 Bone mass and osteoporosis.

change becoming thinner, with less glycogen activity, higher mean pH and change in bacterial flora in favour of coliforms.

This is seen clinically as the genitourinary syndrome of menopause (GSM), previously termed as atrophic vaginitis, the new term reflects the changes that also affect other oestrogen-sensitive areas including the urethra and bladder. This, apart from vulval and vaginal features outlined above, also include urinary frequency, urgency, increased rates of urinary tract infection (UTI) and development of new incontinence due to loss of the mucosal seal of the urinary sphincter.

7.6 Treatment of systemic symptoms

If treatment is required (POI or symptomatic), systemic symptoms are best treated with systemic therapy.

The two main categories of treatment are hormonal and non-hormonal medications. The routes of hormonal treatments include oral, transdermal, vaginal or intrauterine. Subdermal oestrogen used to be utilised, but high rates of tachyphylaxis (escalating dose for similar effect) have largely ceased use.

Contraception should continue in POI unless pregnancy is desired as up to 10% will have intermittent ovarian function and pregnancy can occur, although rare.

In general, hormonal medication, called menopausal hormone therapy (MHT), is most effective for symptom relief and this is safe and suitable for the majority of women.

Hormonal therapy

Systemic hormonal options include oestrogen alone for women who do not have a uterus and oestrogen and progesterone in those who have a uterus (combined MHT). This is because oestrogen stimulates endometrial growth and without

Good practice point

Menopausal hormone therapy is contraindicated in a few groups including women with previous oestrogen receptor-positive breast cancer, endometrial cancer, VTE, severe liver disease and undiagnosed vaginal bleeding. Caution is advised in the presence of multiple vascular risk factors and with active migraine history.

progesterone increases the risk of hyperplasia and endometrial malignancy.

Systemic MHT has two regimens, two main methods of administration and three dose ranges.

The two main combined regimens used are cyclic and continuous. In cyclic regimens, progesterone is given for 14 days in the month on top of daily oestrogen and in continuous regimens, both drugs are given daily. The two main methods of administration are oral and transdermal (intrauterine – Mirena/progesterone only).

Dose ranges are referred by the level of oestrogen component required to relieve symptoms and are low, medium or high dose. The progestogen component is increased or a more potent progestogen is used with higher oestrogen to ensure adequate endometrial protection.

Progesterone forms no other function in MHT and is otherwise kept to a minimum as it is responsible for many of the adverse effects associated with MHT, which include bloating, skin changes and mastalgia and probably most of the small excess in breast cancer risk (worse with oral options and synthetic progestogens).

Oestrogen is also kept to the lowest effective dose for symptom relief as there is no benefit above this. Adverse effects of oestrogen include nausea, vaginal bleeding and dyslipidaemia, a small increase in cholelithiasis, VTE and cardiovascular disease. The latter two are rare and should be balanced against the significant benefits of symptom relief, decreased colorectal cancer and decreased osteoporosis. Transdermal oestrogen is the safest option in terms of VTE and cardiovascular risk and is used in women with risk factors such as hypertension, smoking and obesity or diabetes.

Good practice point

Not all progesterones are the same.

Natural progesterone is extensively and rapidly broken down by first-pass metabolism when given orally; for this reason, either micronized natural or synthetic progestogens are used in MHT.

Norethisterone (NE) is one of the more potent progestogens and is often used with high-dose MHT. It is also reliably absorbed transdermally unlike all other progestogens, and therefore is the only progestogen in combined MHT patches.

The goal of MHT is relief of menopausal symptoms and control of irregular menstruation. Unscheduled bleeding is often poorly accepted and best avoided. Overall, an 80–90% reduction in symptoms is expected.

Women who are within 12 months of the menopause are treated with a cyclic regimen where progestogen is given for 14 days of the month to cause a predictable menstrual bleed and avoid the development of hyperplasia. They can also have continuous progestogen with an intrauterine system (Mirena), if amenorrhoea is preferred, but other forms of continuous progesterone are not suitable due to a high rate of unscheduled bleeding.

Women who are >12 months from their last menstrual bleed can use MHT continuously. This is because they have a greater degree of endometrial atrophy and are less likely to have unscheduled bleeding and usually achieve amenorrhoea.

Oral, transdermal and other options are summarised below in **Table 7.3**.

The risks and benefits of combined MHT (note risks are much lower for oestrogen alone) are summarised below in **Table 7.4**; this is useful when counselling to place risks in real-life understandable context.

Non-hormonal methods

These include complimentary therapies and medications which decrease vasomotor symptoms (VMS) by action on the central nervous system to stabilise adrenergic output and other agents whose mechanism of action is not

> ### Clinical insight
>
> Endometrial ablation is a simple minimally invasive treatment for menorrhagia, however, it does not reliably completely destroy all endometrial tissue. For this reason, women who have had a prior endometrial ablation must have a progestogen included in their MHT to avoid hyperplasia and malignancy in residual endometrium. An intrauterine system is not suitable for this use, as the cavity is scarred and distorted.

> ### Clinical insight
>
> Women with endometriosis who have had a hysterectomy require a progestogen if they have known extra-uterine disease, as otherwise this tissue grows unopposed, which can cause pain and symptomatic masses.

Drug	Oral	Transdermal	Intrauterine
Oestrogen	• Combined equine oestrogen* • Oestradiol valerate* • Oestradiol – Low dose – Medium dose – High dose • Selective oestrogen receptor modulator (bazedoxifene – given in combination product with oestradiol, does not need additional progestogen) – Low dose	• N/A • N/A • Patches/Gel • N/A	N/A for all
Progestogen	• Dydrogesterone (low potency) • Micronized natural progesterone (low potency) • Medroxyprogesterone acetate (MDPA) (moderate potency) • Drospirenone (potent) • NE (potent)	• N/A • N/A • N/A • N/A • In combined patches – Low dose OE – Medium dose OE	Mirena (levonorgestrel IUS) – potent
Other	Tibolone (oestrogenic/ progestogenic/ androgenic actions)	N/A	N/A

*Not used in combined regimens, oestradiol is used in combined regimens.
(IUS, intrauterine system; N/A, not applicable; NE, norethisterone)

Table 7.3 Menopause hormonal therapy options

yet completely understood. All prescribed/non-complimentary therapies have trial data to support efficacy and few, if any, complimentary therapies do.

Women who cannot have systemic oestrogen can use non-hormonal methods. Realistic counselling is important as these on

Risk or benefit	Chance of event per 10,000 women in 1 year using combined MHT compared with non-users	Comparable real-life chance per 10,000 women in 1 year (examples)
Pulmonary embolus	+9	1 in 10,000 = Risk of death in a road traffic crash 10 in 10,000 = Risk of needing emergency hospital treatment for injury from a can or glass over a year
Cardiovascular event (stroke and heart attack)	+15	
Breast cancer	+9	Background lifetime risk is already 1:8 women. High survival
Hip fracture	−6	
Colorectal cancer	−6	
Endometrial cancer	−1	
All-cause mortality	−1 (because most PE and CVD events do not cause death)	
Transdermal oestrogen is not associated with an increase in VTE and probably CV events. Micronised and IU progesterone also confers a significantly lower risk of breast cancer and VTE than oral formulations.		
(CVD, cardiovascular disease; MHT, menopausal hormone therapy; PE, pulmonary embolism; VTE, venous thromboembolism)		

Table 7.4 Risks and benefits of menopause hormone therapy

average provide about half the symptom relief as oestrogen; however, this may be enough to restore quality of life.

Options are outlined below in **Table 7.5** with initiation tips and cautions/side effects/contraindications.

There is reasonable evidence that mindfulness-based therapies such as cognitive

Clinical insight

The cause of VMS is due to sudden alterations in vascular tone at the skin caused by changes in the activity of the thermoregulatory zone of the hypothalamus in response to low oestrogen and high FSH. Sudden superficial vasodilatation leads to loss of heat through the skin surface, characteristic rapid flushing and the sensory experience of feeling hot.

Drug	Mechanism	Initiation	Cautions
Selective noradrenaline reuptake inhibitors • Venlafaxine • Desvenlafaxine Usually does not require 'full' antidepressant dose, with good effect seen at half this. SE, therefore, usually mild	Inhibition of autonomic adrenergic stimulus from hypothalamus, reduction in skin vasodilatation and hot flushes	• Start at one quarter to one half treatment dose (37.5 mg VF). Allow 2 weeks for response • Extended-release preparation available (desvenlafaxine) • Avoid taking dose at night	• Nausea and anxiety with initiation • Do not stop suddenly – taper off (discontinuation symptoms) • Monitor BP at full dose • ↑Insomnia • ↑Sexual dysfunction
Centrally-acting alpha receptor antagonist • Clonidine	• Inhibition of central adrenergic output • Modest effect – 10–20% reduction	Start at 25 mg, increase to one tablet, if tolerated Abandon, if no response at 100 mg/day (two tablets)	• Hypotension • Dizziness • Sedation
GABA • Gabapentin	Not well understood Probably most effective non-hormonal agent for VMS – at higher doses can be as effective as oestrogen	Take at night, 300 mg, allow 2 weeks for effect, maximum dose for VMS 900 mg in divided doses	• Sleepiness • Dizziness • Taper off, if ceasing (discontinuation syndrome)
St John's wort	• Possible mild antidepressant effect • No effect on VMS		Many interactions – caution. Preferable to initiate standard antidepressant

Table 7.5 Non-hormonal treatment options for menopausal symptoms. *Continues opposite*

Drug	Mechanism	Initiation	Cautions
Vitamin E	• Not well understood • May have some effect		Safe
Soy	Oestrogenic effects – may help VMS		Also contra-indicated in women who have a CI to oestrogen
Other herbals • Black cohosh (BC) • Red clover • Wild yam • Omega-3 • Evening primrose	No convincing evidence of effect in well-conducted trials. Available OTC. Women with mild symptoms may prefer to use these after counselling and are likely to do well on them as symptoms already minor		BC is associated with idiosyncratic liver toxicity and other safety concerns

(BP: blood pressure; GABA: gamma-aminobutyric acid; OTC: over-the-counter; SE: side effects; VF: venlafaxine; VMS: vasomotor symptom)

Table 7.5 *Continued*

Guiding principle

Natural, herbal and over-the-counter products are often considered by women to be inherently safe and superior to prescribed drugs. Many therapies are ineffective, but without harmful effects however both major interactions and harm can occur.

Always specifically ask in your medication history if the woman also takes any 'herbal, complimentary or other over-the-counter medications including creams, drops and puffers'. This provides a good opportunity to discuss the reasons for their use and address health beliefs and provide positive education.

behavioural therapy are helpful in adjustment to symptoms, as is a healthy lifestyle and exercise. Compounded bioidentical therapies are not recommended as it is safer to use proprietary medications.

7.7 Treatment of genital symptoms

The genital syndrome of menopause, discussed above, responds well to local topical therapies. It will also respond to systemic therapies; however, the small additional risks to the woman of systemic oestrogens are not warranted to treat genital symptoms alone. The two main treatment options are hormonal, with vaginal oestrogen, or non-hormonal, with vaginal hydrators.

Many breast cancer survivors can have vaginal oestrogen, but many high-grade or advanced-stage endometrial cancers are not recommended to do so – this is because the most common site of recurrence for endometrial cancers is in the vaginal vault. Breast cancer metastases tend to be distant to the vagina and systemic absorption from topical oestrogens is minimal. Additionally, trial data does not show an increased risk of recurrence in breast cancer survivors who use vaginal oestrogen, but there is no good quality data for high-grade endometrial and some ovarian malignancies that express oestrogen receptors; therefore, recommendations are made based on first principles for these populations.

Clinical insight

Nearly all women can have vaginal oestrogen safely; the only exceptions are where a woman has had an oestrogen receptor-positive cancer where oncological advice recommends avoiding it. Always discuss such women with their oncologist.

Good practice point

Topical oestriol is theoretically preferred as it has even less effect on endometrial and distant oestrogen receptors than oestradiol.

Hormonal

Vaginal oestradiol or oestriol is used in a loading regimen daily for 2 weeks then two to three times a week for ongoing symptom control and is available in cream or pessary formulation. At this dose the endometrium is not affected and a progestogen is not required.

Non-hormonal

Non-hormonal options include Replens and other proprietary vaginal hydrators and vaginal lubricants for coitus. Topical oils such as almond oil can provoke cutaneous food sensitisation and newer data suggests that this should be avoided. Other oils such as coconut oil and pawpaw ointment are definite genital irritants and should also be avoided.

Pelvic organ prolapse and urinary dysfunction

chapter 8

8.1 Introduction

The perineum, the area containing the female external genital anatomy (Chapter 1), is the outlet of the largest potential hernial orifice in the body and is under lifetime gravitational stress. Protection from herniation of the pelvic organs is provided by the musculature of the pelvic floor and overlying facia.

Injury due to stretch and avulsion from bony attachment in vaginal childbirth combined with later collagen changes related to age, genital tract atrophy, and menopause and the effects of constipation, straining, coughing and obesity lead to clinically detectable prolapse through this portal and into or beyond the vagina in up to half of parous women.

For this reason, the lifetime risk of prolapse surgery is 11% and one-fifth of elective gynaecology surgeries are prolapse cases.

As prolapse is a common cause of discomfort, functional impairment, urinary and defecatory difficulties with quality of life effects, it is important to have a working understanding of one of the most common problems in adult gynaecology.

8.2 Clinical scenario

A 67-year-old gravida 4, para 4 attends the emergency department for review as she has been unable to void urine for 12 hours and has significant suprapubic discomfort. She reports a long history of a vaginal lump which rubs on her underwear and which she has at times manually reduced for comfort or to help empty her bladder, although it always recurs. She is otherwise systemically well and has no other symptoms of relevance such as fever, dysuria, haematuria, flank pain or abdominal masses.

Background conditions include hypertension, obesity with a body mass index (BMI) of 42 kg/m^2 and type two diabetes on metformin without end-organ complications. She denies post-menopausal bleeding and is not sexually active.

Examination shows an uncomfortable looking obese woman with normal vital signs. There is suprapubic tenderness and genital examination shows a cystocoele (bladder prolapse) to below the hymen, which feels tense.

Diagnostic approach

This case is a straightforward presentation of acute urinary retention. Possible precipitants from history and examination include worsening prolapse with kinking of the urethra or urinary tract infection (UTI), although the lack of other symptoms makes this less likely. Constipation is not generally a cause of urinary retention in women, unlike men, as the urethra is separated from the rectum by the vagina and less susceptible to compression from impacted faeces.

Clinical investigations

A diagnostic and therapeutic indwelling catheter is inserted with relief of pain and 1.7 L of urine is drained rapidly. Full ward test of the catheter urine is negative for nitrites, leucocytes and blood making UTI unlikely. A specimen is sent for formal microscopy and culture, as urine dipsticks have an appreciable false-negative rate.

Creatinine and electrolytes are normal on haematological investigation. No further tests are indicated in initial management.

Management

The woman is admitted overnight for observation and catheter education. She is fitted with a leg bag and taught how to empty this regularly. An urgent appointment is made in the urogynaecology clinic to discuss the options of vaginal pessary or surgery and a 'trial of void' after reduction and/or a week of bladder rest.

An immediate trial of void is avoided as the high urine volume and ongoing prolapse make it likely to fail, as the bladder is both poorly contractile from chronic overstretch and has outlet obstruction at the urethra due to prolapse.

8.3 Pelvic organ prolapse

Pelvic organ prolapse refers to prolapse of the bladder, rectum or cervix into the lower vagina or beyond the hymen.

This causes symptoms due to mass effect from the lump, alteration in the position of pelvic viscera and difficulty with urinary, defecatory and sexual function. Many women do not report symptoms, sometimes despite quite objectively severe prolapse. Importantly, as recurrence is common and repeat surgery is more complicated, operations are only performed for women with bothersome symptoms, which justify surgical repair and these risks.

Types

There are three main areas affected by pelvic organ prolapse (POP), these are often termed 'compartments' (**Figure 8.1**) They are:

1. The anterior compartment, composed of anterior vaginal wall, with descensus of the bladder into the vagina as a cystocoele
2. The posterior compartment, composed of posterior vaginal wall, with descensus of the rectum into the vagina as a rectocoele
3. The apical compartment composed of cervix (or vaginal vault, if the woman has had a previous hysterectomy); this prolapses directly into the vaginal canal

Pathophysiology and epidemiology

The pelvic floor, composed of levator muscles, fascial covering and intact neurological innervation, prevents prolapse due to inherent strength in the tissues and tonic basal muscular contraction.

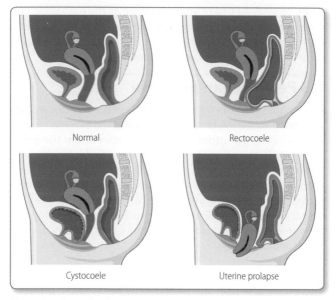

Figure 8.1 Types of prolapse.

Prolapse occurs due to any combination of pelvic floor tissue injury, age and menopause-related loss of tissue collagen, increased load from above and neurological injury. Common causes of pelvic floor injury include:

- Vaginal childbirth, especially repeated births, if the baby is large or forceps are required. This is because in vaginal birth the levator muscles and fascia are stretched and can exceed their tensile strength as well as tear or avulse from bony attachments to the pubic bone and pelvic wall. The tissue supporting the vaginal walls (fascia) is also permanently stretched
- Menopause, because this causes the oestrogen receptor containing tissues of the vaginal walls and pelvis to lose collagen and their inherent strength
- Obesity, chronic cough and constipation because this increases the weight the pelvic floor must resist to avoid prolapse

- Neurological problems or injury such as pudendal nerve neuropathy from prolonged labour, congenital lesions in spina bifida and acquired lesions in spinal cord injury because this impairs the ability of the muscles to contract and resist herniation

Of the above factors, the most prevalent is vaginal childbirth. The relative risk or prolapse is 4 after one birth and 11 after four births.

Clinical features

Clinical features of prolapse are described by site (anterior/posterior/apical) and severity.

Prolapse site

The clinical features of the various types of prolapse are summarised in **Table 8.1**.

Prolapse stages

Prolapse is also classified into stages reflecting severity. Unfortunately for the novice practitioner, there are several classification systems in common use and this can cause confusion when directly comparing prolapse severity.

While a learning practitioner in gynaecology is not expected to describe a prolapse in significant detail and a general description of the site and appearance is adequate, those who wish to learn a system are encouraged to use the 'Pelvic Organ Prolapse Quantification (POP-Q)' system, as this measures the prolapse in standardised sites in centimetres in a standardised way. This is pictured in **Figure 8.2**.

Diagnostic approach

The diagnosis of prolapse is based on a typical history of symptoms as in **Table 8.1** and/or lump identified by the woman and examination consistent with prolapse.

Prolapse examination

Examination of prolapse involves gravity and is different to other components of a gynaecological examination you have previously learned – this is because prolapse itself is

Types	Symptoms	Signs	Complications
Anterior compartment – bladder prolapses with anterior vaginal wall into the lower vagina	• *Urinary:* Symptoms of obstructed urination, incomplete voiding (urethra kinked), need to elevate prolapse digitally to void and frequent voiding • *General:* Sensation of lump or bulge, worse at end of day, ache, dragging, rubbing and vaginal skin irritation • *Sexual:* Pain, discomfort and coital urinary incontinence	Visible bulge in anterior lower vagina or beyond the hymen*	Urinary retention (acute and painful) and urinary retention (chronic and painless) with hydronephrosis and renal injury
Posterior compartment – rectum prolapses with posterior vaginal wall into the lower vagina	• *Bowel:* Symptoms of obstructed defecation, constipation, needing to digitally reduce prolapse to use bowels and general as for anterior compartment • *Sexual:* Pain and discomfort	Visible bulge in posterior lower vagina or beyond the hymen	Constipation
Apical – cervix (or vaginal cuff, if prior hysterectomy) prolapses into lower vagina	Lump at introitus + General symptoms + Sexual symptoms – pain/dyspareunia	Visible central bulge	
Complete (all three compartments, also called a procidentia)	Can have general sexual and bladder/bowel symptoms as per specific compartments above depending on degree of prolapse and bladder/bowel involvement	Everted vagina, cervix leading and 'sock' appearance**	

* All prolapse increases with Valsalva.
** All types have the potential complication of skin injury, erosion and ulceration, this is more common with severe prolapse.

Table 8.1 Prolapse signs and symptoms by compartment affected

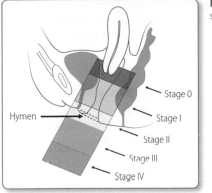

Figure 8.2 Prolapse stages.

Stage 0

Hymen

Stage I

Stage II

Stage III

Stage IV

dynamic and changes in apparent severity with standing and straining.

Complete a general, abdominal, vulval and bimanual examination, as this will demonstrate most moderate and severe prolapse sites and allow you to also identify the size and mobility of the uterus. If the prolapse is outside the body, gently reduce it with lubricated gloved fingers. Ask the woman to bear down and record the maximum severity of the prolapse in this position and take note of the degree of descent of the anterior vaginal wall, posterior vaginal wall and cervix. If your examination is normal and you are not able to identify prolapse, ask the woman to stand and then repeat bearing down to demonstrate her prolapse.

Insert two-gloved fingers in the vagina and ask the woman to squeeze in as if holding her bladder and assess both the subjective strength of the muscles and duration of contraction sustained. Palpate the attachments of the levator ani to the underside of the pubic ramus by turning your finger pulp upwards and feeling each side of the urethra, avulsion from the ramus from childbirth is felt as an absence of muscle and presence of smooth bony edge and can be unilateral or bilateral. Avulsions and descent on Valsalva beyond the hymen are associated with more severe prolapse, a higher risk of recurrence with treatment and failure of physiotherapy.

Finally, perform a speculum examination and examine the walls of the vagina, loss of normal rugae is common at sites of prolapse and reflects damaged vesico-vaginal and recto-vaginal fascial tissue.

Investigations

Minimal investigations are required. If you suspect urinary retention, exclude this with a renal tract ultrasound. If prolapse is sudden, also arrange pelvic ultrasound to exclude new abdominal mass or ascites causing this effect – this is rare, but serious if missed.

Women having surgical treatment should also have a mid-stream specimen of urine (MSU) to assess for concomitant UTI. She should also have a pelvic ultrasound to assess for uterine size, mobility, endometrial thickness and presence of ovarian pathology, as a thickened endometrium requires curettage to exclude hyperplasia/malignancy, a large uterus or unexpected fibroid may not be suitable for vaginal hysterectomy, and ovarian pathology requires a different surgical approach.

Management

The two broad management options for prolapse are non-surgical and surgical.

Non-surgical treatments are preferred where prolapse is mild (above the hymen), symptoms are mild or the woman is not fit for, or declines, surgical management.

Surgical treatments are indicated with more severe prolapse (at the level of the hymen or below) in women who request surgical intervention. There is an up to 40% lifetime re-operation rate, as most surgery is done with native tissue, meaning the stretched prolapse tissue is reinforced and further failure of this tissue is possible. Mesh was previously commonly used for this reason and has lower recurrence rates; however, it had an up to 10% risk of long-term major complications including pain, scarring and migration. Removal is technically difficult and may not fix mesh-related pain. Because of this, the use of mesh has largely ceased.

Non-surgical treatments

These include weight loss, pelvic floor physiotherapy, vaginal pessaries and vaginal oestrogen therapy.

Pelvic floor physiotherapy increases the strength of the levator muscle to reduce symptoms of prolapse, as a stronger muscle is more able to resist pressure from intra-abdominal contents and increases in intra-abdominal pressure. Physiotherapy is no longer effective alone when the prolapse is more severe (hymen or below), as the fascial tissues and muscles are too stretched to meaningfully resist the prolapse of abdominal organs.

Pessaries are inert silicone devices placed in the vagina to elevate the prolapse. They are changed twice a year and require the use of vaginal oestrogen in post-menopausal women to reduce the risk of erosion/injury to vaginal mucosa. There are two main types in common use: (1) ring pessaries, which are generally effective for milder prolapses and (2) Gellhorn pessaries, which have a solid base and can support more severe prolapse (**Figure 8.3**). Motivated women can generally insert and remove their own ring pessary and coitus is possible with

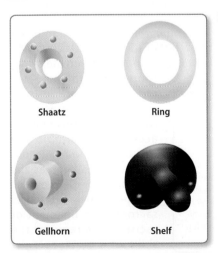

Figure 8.3 Pessary types.

Shaatz

Ring

Gellhorn

Shelf

a ring in situ, but a Gellhorn pessary requires a gynaecologist to exchange and does not permit penetrative sex.

Surgical treatments

Surgical treatments for prolapse are grouped into non-obliterative and obliterative procedures. Non-obliterative procedures are further subdivided into anterior, posterior and apical repairs. In non-obliterative procedures, the aim is to reduce prolapse in the affected compartment and in obliterative procedures, the vagina is permanently closed.

The procedure with the highest success rate and lowest chance of recurrence is colpocleisis, this is obliterative. As colpocleisis is fast and can be performed under spinal anaesthesia, it is the procedure of choice for frail women who will never be sexually active in the future, who are not fit for major surgery and have failed or declined pessary therapy.

In non-obliterative procedures, as prolapse surgery is performed in the affected vaginal compartment, careful pre-operative examination is used to advise the correct procedure. This can either be stand-alone, e.g. anterior repair, if only one compartment has prolapsed, or in combination, e.g. anterior and posterior repair and vaginal hysterectomy/vault suspension, if multiple compartments are affected.

It is important to note that when there is significant descent of the cervix, the defect of apical vaginal supporting mechanisms needs to be properly corrected; otherwise, symptoms (and prolapse) will remain after anterior/posterior repair and traditional hysterectomy. This requires accessing a suitable site to suspend the top (vault) of the vagina such as the intra-peritoneal uterosacral ligaments, extra-peritoneal sacrospinous ligament or sacrum. This requires the skills of a gynaecologist

> ### Good practice point
>
> Women can be inhibited in demonstrating the true extent of their prolapse when examined awake and often prolapse is noted to be more severe under general anaesthetic. For this reason, if you are uncertain about which compartments will need operating in addition to your primary site, it is best to discuss the possibility of all with the woman and consent for this pre-operatively.

with specific training in pelvic floor surgery such as an urogynaecologist.

Discharge the woman on post-operative day 2–3 when her pain is controlled, she can mobilise comfortably, her bladder is functioning normally and she feels able to cope. Provide a prescription for short-term pain relief, sparing opioids if possible (as they are both sedating and constipating) and aperients. Advise all women of post-operative instructions including symptoms of infection, avoidance of heavy lifting, straining, constipation and advice regarding perineal care with good hygiene and sitz baths. Nothing should be inserted into the vagina until primary surgical healing has occurred, in practise this is at 6 weeks.

8.4 Urinary incontinence

Urinary incontinence affects around one-third to one-half of all women during their lifetime and is often not disclosed, unless enquired due to embarrassment. Faecal incontinence is less common at around 3–5%, but even more taboo. Both predominantly affect women and are associated with child-bearing through either direct sphincteric overstretch, perineal tearing, neurological injury or by creating hypermobility of the bladder neck due to prolapse.

To understand incontinence, the mechanisms that normally maintain continence need to be grasped.

Normal continence

Normal continence is achieved by co-operation of the bladder, urethra, pelvic floor muscles and adequate mobility to void at a desired time. Put simply, urine will leak when the pressure inside the bladder exceeds the pressure of the urinary sphincter and problems with bladder storage, urethral contraction and pelvic floor function can cause this to occur non-voluntarily.

In general, the sympathetic nervous system aids continence by keeping the bladder relaxed and internal urinary sphincter contracted. This favours filling at low pressures. The parasympathetic system aids voiding by contracting the bladder and relaxing the internal urethral sphincter at the desired time.

The sympathetic system uses the hypogastric nerve and the parasympathetic system uses the pelvic nerve.

Voluntary control also exists via the pudendal nerve and women can delay voiding by contracting the voluntary external urethral sphincter and their pelvic floor, as when searching for a bathroom when the need to void is great!

Bladder

The bladder needs to able to remain relaxed and store urine until full and then contract and void at a suitable time emptying fully.

During the filling phase, sympathetic input dominates via the hypogastric nerve and keeps the bladder dome relaxed by inhibiting detrusor contraction.

During the voiding phase this inhibition is withdrawn and parasympathetic stimulation via the pelvic nerve causes detrusor contraction.

Urethra

The urethra needs to be protected from increase in intra-abdominal pressure forcing urine out, but also allow free flow of urine when voiding is desired. This is performed by action of the pelvic floor muscles (below) and by contraction of the involuntary (internal) and voluntary (external) urethral sphincter muscles.

During filling, the sympathetic nervous system contracts the involuntary internal sphincter and increases voluntary external sphincter tone. The voluntary sphincter can also be deliberately contracted at times of additional stress (e.g. jumping or coughing) to avoid leakage.

Clinical insight

During voiding, the parasympathetic nervous system inhibits sympathetic outflow to the involuntary sphincter via the pelvic nerve and also inhibits pudendal nerve outflow to the voluntary sphincter; this is why it get very hard to defer voiding when the bladder is very full, as parasympathetic signals to void become stronger in proportion to stretch.

Pelvic floor muscles

The pelvic floor muscles need to be able to support the bladder in a normal position, resist rises in intra-abdominal pressure and relax when void-ing is desired. This occurs partly due to natural resting tone and reflexively with coughing and sneezing, but can be aug-mented by voluntary contraction of the component muscles, collectively called the levator ani, via the pudendal nerve. This causes elevation of the bladder and compression of the urethral sphincter aiding continence.

Pathophysiology and epidemiology

The main forms of urinary incontinence you will encounter are stress incontinence (leaking with increased intra-abdominal pressure such as jumping, sneezing and coughing) and urinary urgency with or without urge incontinence (sudden need to urinate and inability to defer this need with or without actual leak).

Stress incontinence is caused by injury to the supports of the bladder neck or urethral sphincter with childbirth and by the same aetiological factors that cause prolapse, namely age, menopause, obesity and chronic cough. It predominates in reproductive-aged women and older women.

Urgency and urge incontinence have different aetiologies and in many cases a precise cause is not identified with 90% being idiopathic. The remaining 10% are neurogenic and this group will have identifiable neurological disease. Urgency is associated with UTI, bladder irritants such as caffeine, neuro-logical diseases, diabetes, age and post-menopausal status.

Other forms of incontinence exist including overflow, where the bladder leaks, as it is too full (much like a filled bath eventu-ally leaks over the sides) and functional, where the woman is incontinent as she is physically unable to access a bathroom in a timely fashion due to disability.

History, examination and investigations (including urodynamics)

History

History is grouped into storage, voiding and irritative symptoms and a bladder intake-output diary. It aims to differentiate the two main groups of incontinence.

Also, take a history of risk factors and of foods/medications that can precipitate incontinence, as this helps to solidify your diagnosis and suggest initial treatment steps. For stress incontinence, these are vaginal birth (particularly of large babies or with forceps), associated prolapse, post-menopausal status, angiotensin-converting enzyme inhibitors (causes chronic cough) and diuretics (increased urine production). For urgency, these include nulliparity, post-menopausal status, prior pelvic surgery, neurological problems (stroke, diabetes, Parkinson's disease, dementia and spinal), caffeine and alcohol consumption.

Key features in an incontinence history by the most common causes (stress and urgency) are tabulated in **Table 8.2**.

Storage symptoms	Stress incontinence	Urge incontinence
Sudden need to void (urinary urgency): • Typical triggers 'thinking of loo' or 'key in the door' or 'running tap'	• Urgency usually secondary to inability to hold full bladder rather than true urgency • Triggers full bladder, jumping, lifting, etc. • ± Associated urinary leakage (small volume)	• Sudden need to void present • Typical triggers present (key in door, tap running and thinking of loo) • Inability to defer • ± Associated urinary leakage (large volume) 'lose the lot'
Frequency	Usually deliberate in order to reduce risk of leakage from coughing, sneezing, etc.	Usually present and unavoidable due to spontaneous urgency
Leakage with increased abdominal pressure (stress symptoms)	• Present • Dominant feature	• Absent • Non-dominant feature
Nocturia: • Passage of urine >3 times a night	Absent	Present
Continuous leakage	Not a feature – suspect urinary tract fistula or overflow	

Table 8.2 Key features in incontinence history taking. *Continues opposite*

Storage symptoms	Stress incontinence	Urge incontinence
Voiding symptoms		
Incomplete voiding: • **Feeling bladder is not empty at end of void** • **Slow voiding/ difficulty initiating void**	May be present when there is associated prolapse. ± Reducing prolapse digitally to void	Not a feature
Irritative symptoms		
Pain: • **Experienced on bladder filling**	Not a feature unless superimposed urinary tract infection	Can be present, suspect bladder pain syndrome* and diagnosis rather than pure urgency/urge incontinence
Dysuria: • **Experienced on voiding**		Not a feature unless superimposed urinary tract infection
Bladder diary		
Daytime: • **Number of voids, volume, leaks and volume** *Night-time:* • **Number of voids, volume and leaks** *Intake:* • **Water, caffeine and alcohol** • **Recommended intake is 1.5–2 L/day, minimal caffeine (one to two cups) and alcohol**	Empties <8 × day, 300–500 cc voids and leaks with coughing/ sneezing/jumping 0–1 voids, up to 2 if elderly and leaks are uncommon Both types often minimise intake	Empties >8 × day, voids small volumes and urgency ± leaks Nocturia present (>2 × night) and leaks can occur Both types often minimise intake

*Bladder pain syndrome is an uncommon specific diagnosis characterised by pain attributable to the urinary bladder that is associated and worse with filling. This is associated with frequency and urgency. This syndrome is due to mucosal bladder pathology and neurologic adaptation.

Table 8.2 *Continued*

Examination

Examine for associated prolapse, as per the prior section, as this makes stress incontinence more likely and also assess for hypermobility of the bladder neck. This is done by asking the woman to bear down and observing for rotation of the urethral meatus and distal urethra – seen as rotation of the anterior vaginal wall next to the meatus as a direct anatomical relation. The 'Q-tip test,' where a Q tip is placed in the urethra to make this obvious, is rarely used, as it is uncomfortable.

Perform a urinalysis for evidence of UTI (leucocytes and nitrites) and bladder lesions (blood), as UTI and bladder malignancy are both differential diagnoses and at first visit, send a formal mid-stream urine, as this is more reliable than urinalysis at excluding infection.

Assess the integrity of the lower sacral dermatomes and pudendal nerves by performing an assessment of perineal and perianal sensation and myotomes with anal wink to touch and pelvic floor contraction to request. This is helpful where neurological injury is suspected, as this occurs through spinal disease as well as obstetric injury.

Investigations

Investigation of incontinence is grouped into non-invasive and invasive tests. Much useful information is gained with non-invasive tests; however, invasive tests are required to assess the appearance of the bladder lining as well as differentiate objectively between stress incontinence and urge incontinence.

Non-invasive testing Non-invasive testing firstly includes a bladder input-output diary as this gleans useful information regarding voiding volumes, times, symptoms, accidents and consumption of inadequate, excessive or bladder irritant fluids. Memory is often unreliable.

Other non-invasive tests include renal tract imaging for pre-micturition and post-void residual to assess bladder emptying and retention and a uroflow assessment with post-void residual to detect poor stream and retention, respectively.

Uroflow is performed by free void above a calibrated toilet, which records the volume and rate of fluid delivery and can demonstrate abnormally slow voiding or small volume void. An ultrasound performed after voiding will identify if the void is complete or retention is present (post-void residual volume >150 mL).

Invasive testing Invasive testing includes urodynamics and cystoscopy. Urodynamics is a functional assessment of bladder and urethral function. Cystoscopy is a visual assessment of bladder wall appearance, integrity and presence of intravesical pathology.

Urodynamics involves placement of rectal and bladder pressure sensors (**Figure 8.4**) to detect intra-abdominal and intra-vesical pressures after a free uroflow (void). This is followed by sequential steps of measurement of residual

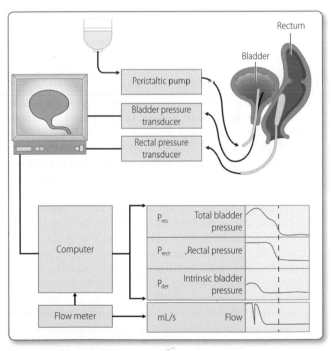

Figure 8.4 Urodynamics.

volume, bladder filling, stress (cough) and urgency (hand-washing and tap) provocative manoeuvres and emptying with continuous measurement of vesical and abdominal pressures, void volume and flow rate. Prolapse is reduced if present and bladder assessment is repeated to detect stress incontinence masked by alteration of the angle of the bladder neck and urethra.

Simultaneous ability to identify bladder and abdominal pressures permits identification of inappropriate detrusor contractions in urge incontinence (an increase in vesical pressure without increase in abdominal pressure is caused by detrusor contraction). It can also detect stress incontinence (an increase in abdominal pressure causing an increase in intra-vesical pressure) and can separate stress incontinence into those caused primarily by urethral neck hypermobility (where high urethral closing pressures are recorded) and intrinsic sphincteric deficiency (where low closing pressures are recorded).

This has implications for treatment options for both the incontinence and associated prolapse. Isolated stress incontinence without prolapse, symptoms of urinary urgency/voiding dysfunction or a history of surgery for prolapse/incontinence is the only clinical presentation where urodynamics are generally not recommended before surgery. Urodynamics is particularly important when severe prolapse exists, as these women have a high rate of occult stress incontinence. Urodynamics can identify which women would benefit from a concurrent anti-incontinence procedure or at least be warned that stress incontinence can develop after surgery.

Cystoscopy is performed while awake with a flexible cystoscope or under anaesthetic with a rigid cystoscope and has several components: Urethral examination, filling, systematic 360° bladder inspection, examination of the trigone and ureteric jets, followed by hydrodistention for 1–2 minutes, emptying under vision and refilling. This identifies intrinsic bladder pathology including transitional cell cancers, cystitis cystica from recurrent UTI, stones, trabeculation from obstructed voiding and glomerulations, haematuria, Hunner's ulceration and a small functional capacity in interstitial cystitis. It is performed where bladder pain, irritation, frequent infection or recurrent haematuria is present to differentiate these conditions.

Urge incontinence management

The management of urinary urgency/incontinence is predominantly conservative or medical and rarely surgical. This is because the problem is primarily neurological and the mainstay of treatment is suppressing inappropriate frequent voiding and retraining neurological responses pharmacologically or behaviourally to achieve more normal bladder habits.

> ### Good practice point
>
> Urinary urgency and urge incontinence, especially when new, should prompt a search for other causes, especially UTI and bladder irritants such as stones and malignancy as well as the presence of neurological disease. This is because these conditions present with similar symptoms and should be individually treated.

Surgery, apart from implantation of sacral nerve stimulators, which are highly specialised, cannot achieve this effect.

Conservative therapies

These consist of bladder training and dietary and lifestyle modification tabulated in **Table 8.3**.

Medical therapies

Medical therapy of urge incontinence consists of use of two major classes of drugs, muscarinic antagonists to inhibit parasympathetically driven detrusor contractions and sympathomimetic agonists to relax the dome. There is also a role for vaginal oestrogen therapy, tricyclic antidepressants and desmopressin. These are tabulated in **Table 8.4**.

Stress incontinence management

The management of stress incontinence is initially conservative, as most cases will improve significantly and this can be adequate to avoid the need for further treatment.

There is a role for surgery in cases who fail to respond or who are severe and are unlikely to respond adequately to conservative treatment alone.

Treatment	Details	Effect
Moderate fluid intake	1.5/L/day	Avoids excess dilute urine (reflex contractions to stretch) or irritant concentrated urine in the bladder (contractions to irritation)
Avoid bladder irritants	Avoid citrus caffeine, alcohol and tea	Less unstable detrusor contractions in response to lower bladder wall stimulation
Bladder training (BT)	Via physiotherapist – training to gradually increase time urine is retained between voids. Starts with short intervals of 1 hour and building to 3–4 hours over weeks to months	• Retrains bladder to tolerate normal volume of urine and gradual downregulation of unstable detrusor contractions • First-line therapy
Biofeedback	Pressure transducers intra-vesical/rectal or electromyogram (EMG) – allows visualisation of detrusor contractions and ability to learn control and inhibition	As for BT above

Table 8.3 Conservative therapeutic options for urinary urgency and urge incontinence

Conservative therapies

This includes a women's health physiotherapist for training in pelvic floor muscle strengthening, as this helps to resist leakage of urine with increase in intra-abdominal pressure.

Supervised exercise is superior to independent exercise in clinical efficacy as a substantial proportion of women do not recruit the correct muscle groups and require real-time feedback to do so successfully and consistently.

Medical therapies

This consists of vaginal oestrogen in post-menopausal women, as this improves urethral mucosal seal by increasing the

Medications	Mechanism of action
Anti-muscarinic drugs:	
• Oxybutynin • Oxytrol	Non-selective and bind to bladder and other muscarinic receptors, blocking detrusor contraction in response to parasympathetic nerve action and release of acetylcholine. They, therefore, have high rates of generalised anti-cholinergic effects including dry mouth, eyes, constipation as well as confusion and worsening of cognitive impairment. The patch or slow-release formulations are better tolerated overall, although there is a 10% skin reaction to patches
• Darifenacin • Solifenacin	More selective for bladder muscarinic receptors and have less generalised anticholinergic effect
• Tolterodine	Tolterodine is non-selective, but has high affinity for the bladder and low affinity for salivary glands and has less anticholinergic undesirable effects than oxybutynin
Tricyclic antidepressants	Mixed action – stimulation of urinary sphincter contraction, bladder analgesia and relaxation of bladder dome
Desmopressin (DDAVP)	Vasopressin analogue, acts on the collecting ducts to increase water resorption and decrease urine formation and, thus, nocturia
Oestrogen	Bladder trigone and urethral oestrogen receptor stimulation in post-menopausal women result in less unstable bladder contractions due to mucosal thickening/ resistance to irritants and greater sphincteric integrity

Table 8.4 Pharmacological therapy for urinary urgency and urge incontinence

volume of cells lining the distal urethra and vagina. Women can also be offered a trial of duloxetine in off-label use as this increases pudendal nerve firing and therefore urinary sphincter tone.

Surgical therapies

Surgical therapies for stress incontinence are minimally invasive or open/laparotomy.

Minimally invasive techniques include mid-urethral sling and laparoscopic Burch colposuspension. Open techniques include Burch colposuspension and autologous fascial sling.

Mid-urethral sling is the most common operation, as it is quick, highly effective (>90% dry), has low complications and is performed as a day surgery. It is important to exclude baseline urinary retention before the procedure, as this will be worsened and permanent intermittent catheterisation required. There is also a 10% risk of new urinary urgency and frequency after mid-urethral sling.

8.5 Recurrent urinary tract infection

This common condition affects 60% of adult women. 10% have at least one UTI per year making it a major cause of morbidity, lost productivity and healthcare expenditure.

Pathophysiology

Women are inherently predisposed to UTI, as the urethra is short and bowel flora is able to traverse the female perineum readily. Sexual intercourse aids this by mechanically disturbing local flora and massaging the urethra where it is adjacent to the anterior vaginal wall aiding the ascent of microorganisms.

Diagnosis

Most women will not have an underlying cause, but all with >3 culture-proven infections in a 12-month period warrant workup to exclude:

- Urinary retention (post-void residual measurement – ultrasound)
- A nidus for microorganisms [consider CT, intravenous pyelo-gram (IVP) or US scan for stone]
- Renal tract malformation (US scan)
- Antibiotic-resistant organism [mid-stream specimen of urine (MSU) antibiotic sensitivity results]

It is important to ensure that other less common bladder pathology such as tumours, stones and bladder pain syndrome as well as other vaginal and pelvic pain conditions also cause similar symptoms to UTI.

This is the reason for mid-stream urine culture 'proof'.

Cystoscopy is a final check to exclude confusable intrinsic bladder pathology, but is not needed in younger women without risk factors for malignancy such as smoking or haematuria.

Management

Advise good urinary hygiene and habits, but avoid condescending information – the majority of adult women are aware of recommended wiping from front to back. Encourage regular bladder emptying, avoiding holding on and ensuring bladder are completely emptied at each void. Also encourage voiding after sex to excrete any bacteria that have ascended during coitus.

Prescribe either low-dose prophylactic antibiotics at night or after sex (depending on the trigger) or a urinary antiseptic (Hiprex). Also prescribe vaginal oestrogen therapy in post-menopausal women, as this decreases infections by improving urethral seal.

Give women a ready request for mid-stream urine and treatment antibiotic to take, if they develop an active infection, so treatment is prompt, as this minimises complications.

Principles of gynaecological oncology

9.1 Introduction

Gynaecological oncology is the sub-specialty area concerned with cancers arising in the female genital tract, i.e. of the uterus, fallopian tubes, ovaries, cervix and vagina. It also includes cancers of the vulva and pregnancy-related malignancy (hydatidiform mole, choriocarcinoma and other gestational neoplasias). Although not a primarily gynaecological organ, gynaecologists also screen for breast malignancy, management is generally under the care of breast surgeons.

Gynaecological cancer is common. Endometrial malignancy, which is driven by obesity, is ever-increasing in incidence however is usually identified at an early stage when it can be cured by surgery, whereas mortality from ovarian cancer continues to be high as this disease is diagnosed stubbornly late, despite much research effort into screening tests.

9.2 Clinical scenario

A 52-year-old para 3 attends due to 6 months of intermittent light non-cyclic vaginal bleeding. She reports no pain, fever or purulent discharge and the bleeding is not post-coital.

Background medical problems include class 3 obesity [body mass index (BMI) 45 kg/m^2], hypertension, type 2 diabetes mellitus (T2DM) and osteoarthritis. She has a surgical history of one caesarean section and takes irbesartan, metformin and paracetamol. There is no history of anticoagulant or hormone replacement use and no medication allergies.

Gynaecologically, cervical screening test (CST) was normal 6 months ago and has never been abnormal. In response to specific questioning, she reports her last menstrual bleed was 18 months ago in the context of prior night sweats and hot flushes. She has never had a sexually transmitted infection (STI) and is in a monogamous relationship and is sexually active without problems with vaginal dryness.

Examination shows a well-appearing obese woman with normal vital signs and a soft abdomen with Pfannenstiel scar. External genitals are unremarkable without blood and speculum examination of the vagina is also unremarkable with a normal cervix.

She asks if her menses should be continuing at her current age.

Diagnostic approach

This is undiagnosed post-menopausal bleeding as there has been >12 months since last menstruation.

Undiagnosed genital tract bleeding has a differential which encompasses uterine, cervical and vaginal sources and causes range from benign to malignant. It should never be dismissed as 'normal' without appropriate investigation.

The prior menopausal transition twelve months before the new bleeding and presence of obesity and diabetes as risk factors for endometrial intraepithelial neoplasia/malignancy point towards this being the most likely cause of the bleeding.

The cervix is unlikely to be the cause due to absence of suspicion for cervicitis (no fever, STI history or high risk exposure) and cervical malignancy (due to normal screening history) and the vagina is also unlikely the cause due to lack of vaginal atrophic change.

Misattribution of urinary or rectal bleeding is unlikely in a physically and cognitively able adult.

Guiding principle

There are many axioms in gynaecology, but one useful rule of thumb is that 'all women are pregnant until proven otherwise and all abnormal bleeding is cancer until proven otherwise.'

This is because missing a pregnancy can cause erroneous care and increase the risk of maternal harm such as from ectopic pregnancy and, although the vast majority of women with abnormal vaginal bleeding do not have cancer, assuming a benign cause without proper investigation will miss some cancers. Late diagnosis is associated with worse outcomes and a higher chance of death from disease.

Pelvis US scan is performed to assess the endometrium.

Further investigations

Pelvic ultrasound shows an anteverted normal sized uterus with an endometrial thickness of 14 mm (normal <4 mm). Cystic change is also reported within the endometrium with vascularity on Doppler assessment. All of these findings are suspicious for malignancy.

Pipelle endometrial biopsy is taken and this shows grade one endometrial adenocarcinoma.

Management

Endometrial adenocarcinoma is diagnosed and staging CT of the chest/abdomen/pelvis is performed to screen for metastatic disease. No metastases are identified and after multidisciplinary team meeting confirms histopathology and suitability for surgical attempt at cure, the woman proceeds to laparoscopic hysterectomy, bilateral salpingo-oophorectomy and pelvic lymph node excision by the gynaecological oncology team.

Final histopathology confirms grade one endometrial adenocarcinoma confined to the uterine body with no significant

> ## Good practice point
>
> The gold standard for diagnosing endometrial pathology is hysteroscopy and curettage, as this allows for direct visual identification of pathology.
>
> In suitable cases when intra-cavity polyps or fibroids are not suspected as these cannot be addressed in an outpatient setting, and where cervical stenosis is not present, outpatient pipelle endometrial biopsy can achieve a rapid diagnosis and avoid delay introduced by the need for theatre access and general anaesthesia.

> ## Clinical insight
>
> Multidisciplinary care is common in most aspects of medicine, but is standard in complex areas where the best choice of action depends on the condensation of imaging, clinical, pathological and tumour factors as occurs in cancer care.
>
> Care in a dedicated cancer unit, along with multidisciplinary planning of treatment, is associated with improved outcomes and superior survival. This is due to accurate case selection for treatment options as well as oncologically-sound surgical technique and the complete package of expert post-surgical care and secondary prevention of anticipatable complications as well as appropriate follow-up.

myometrial invasion, lymphovascular invasion and no signs of extra-uterine disease.

The woman is informed of her favourable prognosis malignancy and is also informed that she does not require adjuvant radiotherapy to the vaginal vault.

She is followed-up regularly by local low-risk protocol and discharged after 5 years without evidence of recurrence.

9.3 Principles of cancer staging and treatment

Staging

All cancers are approached from a similar perspective once diagnosis is made, first establishing the tumour type and biologic aggressiveness (grade) and the degree of spread (stage).

Cancers can spread in several ways including by direct local extension, through blood vessels (haematogenous), through lymphatics and through body cavities.

Each tumour has a different inherent predilection for spread. Ovarian cancer is known for direct peritoneal spread, coating the bowel and omentum in 'cake' with distant disease rare. Cervical cancer, conversely, is known for local invasion through the parametrium on either side of the uterus and to the pelvic side wall.

Staging is either clinical (cervical cancer) or surgicopathological meaning excision as completely as possible including draining lymph nodes and pathological examination (other gynaecological cancers).

Cervical cancer is staged differently because many cases are diagnosed in low-resource settings where advanced testing such as MRI may not be available and also because many women will not have surgery as the shift from surgical management to primary chemo-radiotherapy happens at an early stage in this particular cancer, meaning the majority of women will never receive a surgical procedure to stage their cancer. This, however, has been modified in recent years to allow PET scan and MRI to be considered in assigning a stage where it is available. Other malignancies generally have surgery to both resect as much as possible disease and attempt cure unless the woman is unfit for surgery or has stage four (see below) disease on imaging or pathological testing.

The reason for grading and staging tumours is that this allows comparison of 'like with like' and standardises descriptions, allowing use of clinical protocols based upon clinical trial-derived gold standard treatment for the particular malignancy. It also aids research into future treatments.

The International Federation of Gynaecology and Obstetrics (FIGO) is the standardising body for gynaecological malignancy and a useful resource when new to gynaecological cancer staging.

In general, stage one cancers are confined to the organ of origin, stage two cancers extend beyond the initial organ, stage three cancers have loco-regional spread to adjacent structures or lymph nodes and stage four cancers have disease in distant body parts.

Treatment

The default position is curative intent, where treatment is intended to bring about cure, if possible. Odds of this being ultimately successful decrease with higher grade and more advanced stage.

Most cancers are cured by surgical excision either with pre-surgery treatment with chemotherapy (neo-adjuvant) to shrink disease and render it resectable or post-surgical (adjuvant) treatment with chemo- or radiotherapy.

Surgery facilitates response to adjuvant therapy because resecting the majority of the cancer has several benefits including:

- improved metabolic and nutritional patient status (cancer is a large calorie drain)
- increased chemosensitivity of remaining tumour due to increased cellular division as a response to tumour removal (chemotherapy is best at killing rapidly dividing tissues), and
- improvement in penetration of agents into tumour as relatively hypoxic central tissue is less

Cervical cancer is an exception as cure rates are equivalent for primary chemo-radiotherapy for all but the very earliest of tumours (<1B) with a more favourable side effect profile.

9.4 Human papillomavirus-dependent malignancy (vulva, vagina and cervix)

Infection with human papillomavirus (HPV) is almost ubiquitous and nearly all sexually active women will be exposed.

It is acquired with coitus, particularly penile-vaginal, although it also can be orally transmitted. HPV can infect all of the lower genital tract as well as oropharynx, but has a predilection for causing high-grade dysplasia and malignancy at the squamo-columnar junction of the cervix. It does this by integration of viral oncogenes into the host cell genome, overcoming normal controls on division, differentiation and cell migration.

Other sites are much less likely to generate significant dysplasia or malignancy.

The vast majority of HPV-infected adults clear their infection without being aware, a minority, particularly with high-risk types (16 and 18 in particular) progress to high-grade dysplasia and malignancy without treatment. Cervical screening is designed to identify these pre-cancer changes and intervene in cases of high-grade dysplasia to prevent the development of cancer.

Most junior clinicians will never see a vaginal cancer, may encounter vulval ones and are all familiar with prevention of cervical cancer through screening.

Vaginal and vulval cancer

Vaginal cancer is very rare and almost entirely caused by the presence of HPV infection.

Vulval cancer is more common than vaginal cancer and has two main pathways to disease: (1) HPV-driven and (2) HPV-independent/chronic inflammation. Both are less common than cervical cancer in countries without cervical screening programmes.

Vaginal dysplasia and vaginal cancer

Vaginal cancer develops from the precursor vaginal dysplastic lesion termed as vaginal intra-epithelial neoplasia (VAIN). VAIN can progress from low- to high-grade lesions and high-grade VAIN has a 10% risk of developing invasive disease.

Vaginal cancer composes 1% of gynaecological malignancy, is usually squamous histology and spreads by local extension to the bladder, bowel and loco-regional lymph nodes.

Very rare other forms of vaginal cancer exist including melanoma and clear cell carcinoma as well as metastasis from endometrial and other malignancies; these are seen in tertiary referral centres.

Diagnosis VAIN and early vaginal cancer are asymptomatic and are detected at colposcopy (examination of the lower genital tract with a microscope and application of dilute acetic acid and Lugol's iodine solution), usually in women with an abnormal CST result with presence of oncogenic HPV detected.

Established vaginal malignancy presents with vaginal bleeding, discharge, pain in the pelvis and bladder and bowel symptoms from direct invasion.

Management Low-grade VAIN can be observed by a suitably experienced clinician (as it is uncommon and to ensure correct recognition of high-grade disease), but high-grade VAIN should be treated due to risk of progression as should vaginal cancer.

Treatment selection depends on general health/ co-morbidities, diffuse or focal VAIN, potential for sexual activity and patient preference.

Therapeutic options for VAIN are excision, which is preferable in most cases as

> ### Good practice point
>
> Be cautious in reassuring women with high-grade cytology on CST who have a normal (negative) colposcopy of their cervix. This is because undetected VAIN is a potential cause. There are many cases in the literature of serial treatment of the cervix with excision and finally hysterectomy, all with normal histology, only to have a vaginal cancer diagnosed, having been concealed by the speculum blades all along.
>
> Look at the cervix, and vagina, carefully in all dysplasia patients.

Clinical insight

Acetic acid and Lugol's iodine solution are useful in identification of cervical and vaginal dysplasia as these areas can appear normal to the naked eye.

This is because both have differing uptake by dysplastic tissue and create visible contrast, aiding the clinician in optimal biopsy site. Acetic acid reversibly coagulates cells with high protein content such as dysplastic cells with a high nuclear-to-cytoplasmic ratio and active mitosis, much like cooking an egg opacifies the white. Lugol's iodine solution has the reverse effect as it is taken up poorly by cells with low glycogen content such as dysplastic cells who utilise available glycogen more extensively than normal ones leaving them pale and normal cells dark.

This creates the hallmark 'acetowhite, Lugol's pale' pattern seen in dysplasia at colposcopy.

histology is obtained and can exclude invasive cancer, laser or treatment with imiquimod or 5-flurouracil (5-FU) cream (immune activator and chemotherapeutic agent, respectively). Diffuse disease is a particular challenge, as excision requires vaginectomy, a challenging operation associated with appreciable morbidity and sexual impact; topical 5-FU is used if vaginectomy is not appropriate.

Vaginal cancer is treated by chemoradiation in those with potential cure and palliative therapy in the remainder.

Vulval dysplasia and cancer

Unlike cervical and vaginal dysplasia, vulval dysplasia has two pathological pathways: (1) HPV dependent and (2) HPV independent caused by chronic inflammatory change. The latter is seen in women with vulval skin conditions such as lichen sclerosis and is one of the reasons that good control of lichen is recommended.

Risk is increased by smoking (inhibitory effect on adaptive immune response) and immunosuppression (poor innate ability to mount immune response).

Diagnosis This is achieved by history, examination and investigations. The latter consists of histological (when tumour is the rumour, tissue is the issue!) and imaging to determine tumour size and loco-regional spread.

Enquire regarding pruritis, a lump or sore on the genitals and pain. Many women deny symptoms in early cancer, particularly if frail or obese.

Examine the vulva for irregularity, raised lesions, ulcers or more subtle changes of vulval dysplasia which include texture change and pigment change, as well as changes of lichen sclerosis. Cancer generally arises in pre-existing dysplasia. If an obvious cancer is present, examine this for mobility versus fixedness to underlying bone as well as groin lymph nodes, which are enlarged and hard when metastases are present as spread is primarily by local extension and lymphatic dissemination.

Apply 5% acetic acid to suspected areas and take punch biopsy with local anaesthetic for histology – in cases with obvious tumour, avoid necrotic areas as these are less helpful to achieve diagnosis as pathological assessment of dead tissue is difficult due to autolysis and other changes.

Always follow this with colposcopy, cervical smear and biopsy of cervix if abnormal findings as HPV driven vulval dysplasia and malignancy increases the risk of cervical dysplasia and malignancy as HPV can infect the entire lower genital tract.

Management Management depends on patient factors (comorbidities, frailty and fitness for surgery), tumour factors (stage and surgical resectability) and nodal factors (women with nodal disease are incurable).

Women with early-stage tumours which are surgically resectable without positive draining inguinal lymph nodes on imaging or prior groin node dissection, are treated by wide local excision alone for stage 1a, which is a small tumour with <1 mm invasion as risk of nodal metastases is <1%.

All other surgical candidates are treated by modified radical vulvectomy with or without attempt at reconstruction. This is a procedure with high morbidity including venous thromboembolism (VTE), lymphocoele, infection, breakdown and sexual and psychological dysfunction and is reserved for those most likely to be cured. If the mass is mid-line, bilateral vulvectomy and groin node dissection is required. Lateral masses can be treated with hemi-vulvectomy and ipsilateral lymph node dissection; however, if the ipsilateral groin nodes are positive, a contralateral groin node dissection is subsequently performed due to the chance of contralateral metastases in this group.

Vulval cancer, which is advanced stage with either invasion into urethra, bladder, rectum or fixation to underlying bone with or without positive lymph nodes is generally managed palliatively with radiation to control symptoms of mass, bleeding and pain. Carefully selected good candidates (young and fit) can be offered aggressive surgery (exenteration or resection of affected bladder or rectum, stoma or resection of pubic ramus with mass).

Adjuvant therapy is indicated in women with positive lymph nodes and is given as radiation to the tumour bed and groin nodes.

All women are followed clinically in an oncology unit with history of symptoms of recurrence of local and distant disease, examination of lower genital tract for dysplasia/malignancy and palpation of groin nodes until deemed 'clear' of recurrence by local protocol (typically 5–10 years).

Cervical screening and cancer

The sharp decline in the incidence of cervical cancer in countries with embedded screening programmes is a great public health success story which has been enhanced by improved understanding of the pivotal role of HPV infection in pathogenesis and development of an effective vaccine. Unfortunately worldwide death due to this preventable cancer occurs in women and girls leading to huge waste of life.

The process along the oncogenic 'highway' from infection to low-grade dysplasia, high-grade dysplasia and finally malignancy is a variable one and although the natural history is slow in most women (over a decade from infection to serious disease in those destined to develop this), it is also unpredictable meaning a minority of unfortunate women progress rapidly, the majority clear their infection without sometimes being aware it existed and some women never clear their infection but do not progress over time to high-grade disease.

Of all the oncogenic HPV, types 16 and 18 are associated with the majority (>90%) of cervical cancers and type 16 accounts for >75% alone.

Cervical screening methods

Cervical screening methods vary between countries; there are two broad approaches:
1. Human papillomavirus screening (CST)
2. Cytological screening (Pap screening)

Both require collection of a specimen of exfoliated cells from the cervix by speculum examination and collection with a brush/sampling device. Both also require confirmation of findings in high-risk women with colposcopy.

Human papillomavirus driven screening programmes are more sensitive, as they rely on detection of oncogenic HPV without which significant dysplasia is extremely unlikely and this is becoming the dominant approach. It also does not rely on interpretation of cellular atypia, which has inter-observer variability and is less affected by menses and collection technique, all of which pose problems with cytology primary screening.

A HPV test can also be done blindly as a vaginal self-collected swab which is better than no screening in under-screened women and is more acceptable than speculum examination in this cohort. In all other women, a liquid-based medium is used as this can provide HPV deoxyribonucleic acid (DNA) and cytology result, if needed.

Clinical insight

Colposcopy is a medical procedure where a duckbill speculum is inserted into the vagina and the cervix and vagina are examined with a microscope aided by application of dilute acetic acid and Lugol's iodine solution. Biopsy is taken by punch (approximately 3 mm) of areas that are suspicious for dysplasia.

Key areas to visualise are the cervical transformation zone (TZ), the entire ecto-cervix, fornices and vagina. The TZ, where the ecto cervical glandular cells meet the vagina and undergo squamous metaplasia due to exposure to vaginal acidity, is particularly important as this area is especially vulnerable to HPV infection and development of dysplasia and malignancy. This is much less common in other sites (**Figure 9.1**).

There are three types of TZs: (1) a type one TZ is fully visible, (2) a type two TZ is partially within the cervical canal but visible with manipulation and (3) a type 3 TZ is not visible. Surveillance for dysplasia is therefore, very difficult with a type 3 TZ. Older women and those who have not given birth or who have done so by caesarean are more likely to have a type 3 TZ.

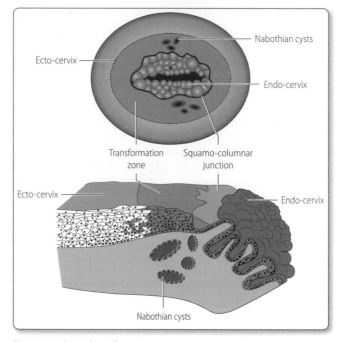

Figure 9.1 Cervical transformation zone.

In HPV screening, screen negative women are reported as low risk without further testing and are rescreened at 5 years. Women who screen positive for oncogenic HPV have automatic cytology performed on the same liquid-based specimen and a report for HPV type and cytology is issued.

In general, high-risk HPV (types 16 and 18) require annual colposcopic examination regardless of reflex cytology result due to the higher risk of dysplasia and intermediate-risk HPV (other types) require colposcopy every 2–3 years unless high-grade cytology is present, as they are significantly less likely to progress or have undetected high-grade dysplasia. Additionally to this, all women with high-grade cytology, regardless of HPV type, require priority colposcopy (<6 weeks), as they are a high-risk population for requiring treatment and for disease progression – this becomes more likely with high-grade than low-grade changes.

In cytology-based screening, otherwise called Pap testing, cervical cytology is collected on a glass slide, fixed and interpreted. Due to limitations listed above, a 10–20% false-negative result and false positives due to inflammation, blood and other non-dysplasia reasons underpin the need for 2 yearly screening.

Low-grade abnormalities HPV type dictates the need for reflex cytology and colposcopy; however, cervical biopsy result dictates management.

This is because severity of dysplasia is defined by the depth of the epithelium affected (superficial, middle third and entire thickness) and to do this accurately requires cells in architecture, achievable by biopsy but not cytology (cells brushed or washed from a surface).

Low-grade abnormalities, equivalent to cervical intraepithelial neoplasia 1 (CIN1), which are usually confirmed by colposcopy and biopsy, unless the risk of occult high-grade disease is low (such as in HPV other and normal or low-grade reflex cytology, which has less frequent colposcopy), are generally observed and not actively treated. This is because the chance of missed high-grade disease is low, the majority of women will clear spontaneously with time and treatment has minor rates of morbidity including bleeding, infection and cervical insufficiency in future pregnancy (rare at 10 mm excision or less).

In certain situations, low-grade abnormalities are treated if agreed upon by patient and clinician including significant patient anxiety, older women with persisting low-grade changes who have completed childbearing, women with

Guiding principle

Cytology and histology give different information. Cytology informs of the nature and dysplastic or malignant features of free-floating cells. This is obtained in cervical screening.

Histology gives tissue in architecture, allowing for not only cellular changes of dysplasia or malignancy to be identified, but also the degree and depth involved, allowing more accurate diagnosis. This is obtained in cervical biopsy.

high-risk HPV and recurrent unsatisfactory colposcopy and where the biopsy is inconsistent with cytology and colposcopy, if both are high grade, especially if type 16 or 18 positive.

Cervical cytology is reported as either normal, low-grade squamous abnormalities [called low-grade squamous intra-epithelial lesion (LSIL)], glandular abnormalities, high-grade squamous abnormalities [called high-grade squamous intra-epithelial lesion (HSIL)] or invasive malignancy.

Cervical biopsy is reported as either normal, presence of inflammation, glandular abnormalities or squamous CIN1, 2 or 3 or malignancy in order of severity. CIN2 and 3 are high-grade disease and should be treated. P16 immunohistochemistry can help to differentiate CIN2, which is likely to progress and merits treatment and is helpful in young women with this finding.

Squamous histology is the most common type of dysplasia and glandular is less common.

High-grade abnormalities High-grade abnormalities encompass a diagnosis of CIN2 or 3 on histopathology of cervical biopsy. They should be treated because the risk of progression to invasive cancer increases, especially with CIN3 where it is 30% and higher with younger women as there is more lifetime risk accumulated.

Treatment options are surgical and include excisional and ablative therapies; there are no medical therapeutic options.

Excisional therapies include electrocautery loop excision, also called large loop excision of the transformation zone ('LLETZ') and cold-knife conisation ('cone biopsy'). Both procedures remove a small portion of cervix and TZ to excise high-grade dysplasia.

A LLETZ loop is used to remove a small segment of outer cervix using diathermy. Conisation involves cutting out a usually slightly larger piece with a knife; this leaves precise histology at surgical margins, as diathermy is not used for removal of the specimen (**Figure 9.2**).

Conisation is performed where either glandular abnormalities are present, the upper edge of the dysplasia is not visible (e.g. type 3 TZ) or where invasive cancer is suspected. This is

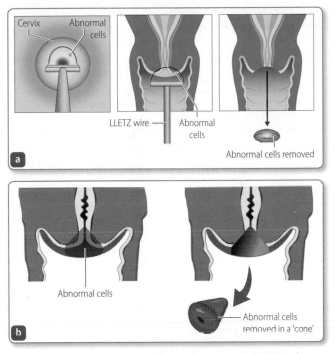

Figure 9.2 (a) Large loop excision of the transformation zone (LLETZ) and (b) cold-knife conisation ('cone biopsy').

because the status of the margins for dysplasia is clear due to absence of diathermy effect in the specimen (cut with a knife not electrocautery). This is also the reason the specimen is usually larger.

All other women are offered a LLETZ and this is the more common procedure; diathermy artefact at the margins is reduced by good technique.

Ablative procedures include laser and cryotherapy; women must be carefully selected for suitability with appropriate biopsy and fully visible disease without any suspicion of cancer, as no histology is obtained to exclude an early cancer.

All women are followed-up with a test of cure for their HPV/dysplasia. This entails repeat cervical screening at 1 and 2 years with HPV DNA and cytology until clear on two occasions.

Post-coital bleeding

Post-coital bleeding is a red flag symptom (meaning potential malignancy as a cause) and implies bleeding from the cervix with mechanical contact.

Possible causes include benign pathology including cervicitis from non-sexually and STIs as well as ectropion, polyps and, finally, malignancy. This is most women's fear, but the least common cause.

Key history, examination and investigation steps are outlined in **Table 9.1**.

Most women are diagnosed correctly clinically in combination with biopsy and swabs.

Infection is treated with appropriate antibiotics, full STI screening and sexual partner contact tracing, cervical polyps are excised, and high-grade dysplasia treated by excision (see above section). Cancer is referred for oncological care.

	Items	Significance
History	• Duration and heaviness of bleeding	• Heavy bleeding more concerning for sinister pathology • Longer duration – greater risk of complications or progression
	• Risk factors for STI (new partner, multiple partners, prior STI and other symptoms)	• Cause more likely to be infective
	• Risk factors for cervical cancer (no HPV vaccination, age, sexual partners, no barrier contraception, smoking and history of abnormal screening)	• Chance of cervical cancer as cause
	• Hormonal medication use	• Chance of bleeding related to breakthrough atrophic bleeding
	• Pattern of the bleeding (post-coital vs. inter-menstrual)	• Inter-menstrual bleeding more commonly associated with endometrial cause, post coital cervical cause
Examination	• Speculum – cervical appearance	• Can visually identify cervicitis, ectropion, polyps and cancer 1B+. Permits swabs and co-test collection for diagnosis
	• Colposcopy of cervix	• Identifies areas suspicious of dysplasia and permits biopsy
Investigation	• Chlamydia, gonorrhoea, mycoplasma, and trichomonas PCR swab	• Identify STI cervicitis
	• Endocervical MCS swab	• Identify non-STI cervicitis
	• Co-test of cervix	• Identify cervical neoplasia and malignancy
	• Biopsy of cervix	
	• Ultrasound of uterus	• Identify polyps and endometrial pathology
(HPV, human papillomavirus; MCS, microscopy, culture and sensitivity; PCR, polymerase chain reaction; STI, sexually transmitted infection)		

Table 9.1 Assessment of post-coital bleeding

Ectropion is a diagnosis of exclusion after co-test and swabs are negative and this is treated by cautery with silver nitrate or diathermy.

Cervical cancer

Cervical cancer is the end point of a minority of high-risk HPV infections, usually over more than a decade. Cancer without HPV is exceedingly rare.

Pathophysiology Cervical cancer is most commonly squamous in histology (80%); other types include adenocarcinoma (most of remainder) and rare subtypes include neuroendocrine, metastatic and melanoma.

Spread of disease occurs primarily by local extension laterally through the parametrium (tissue on either side of the cervix) as well as inferiorly into the vagina, anteriorly into the bladder, posteriorly into the rectum and to the pelvic side wall.

Metastasis also occurs to loco-regional lymph nodes, in particular the pelvic lymph nodes, and para-aortic lymph nodes, if pelvic nodes contain disease.

Diagnosis It is important to note that post-coital bleeding is a late, not an early symptom.

Key clinical features and investigations are outlined in **Table 9.2**.

9.5 Uterine cancers

Uterine cancers are the second common gynaecological cancers comprising endometrial and uterine muscle cancers. Endometrial adenocarcinoma makes up the great majority (>95%). This is because endometrial adenocarcinoma is fuelled by high oestrogen/no progesterone environments, which includes obesity, chronic anovulation [polycystic ovarian syndrome (PCOS)] and low rates of childbearing and lactation. This storm of risk is common in developed nations. Obesity and chronic exposure to endogenous oestrone without the protective effects of ovulation and menstruation explains the post-menopausal presentation in many women.

	Item	Significance
History	• Sensation of mass in pelvis and pelvic pain	• Large tumour
	• Post-coital bleeding	• Bleeding from unstable vessels on tumour surface
	• Watery offensive discharge	• Necrotic tumour
	• Flank pain	• Obstructive hydronephrosis from direct lateral extension of tumour into ureters
	• Leg oedema	• Obstruction of lymphatic drainage from lower limb from lateral tumour spread
	• Haematuria and haematochezia	• Invasion of cancer into bladder and bowel
Examination	• Abdominal examination	• Flank pain from obstructive hydronephrosis
	• Lower limb examination	• Pitting oedema from lymphatic obstruction
	• Loco-regional lymph nodes	• May have palpable enlarged inguinal nodes in late disease
	• Genital examination	• Offensive smelling bloody discharge
	• Speculum examination	• Visible tumour and can extend into the upper vagina
Investigation: • Histopatho-logical	• Cervical biopsy • Cervical cone biopsy/conisation	• Gives histological diagnosis
• Imaging	• CT ± PET	• Can identify tumour size, suspect lymph node metastases on size or PET avidity
	• MRI	• Can identify tumour more precisely and relationship to surrounding structures
	• IVP	• Identifies ureteric obstruction from advanced disease
• Clinical	• Sigmoidoscopy • Cystoscopy	• Identify bladder and bowel invasion from advanced disease
(IVP, intra-venous pyelogram; PET, positron emission tomography)		

Table 9.2 Targeted gynae-oncological assessment

Clinical insight

The pre-malignant lesion for endometrial cancer is endometrial hyperplasia with cellular atypia, also called endometrial intra-epithelial neoplasia. Hyperplasia with atypia has a 30% risk of occult malignancy and is treated in the same manner for this reason.

Other risk factors include the use of unopposed oestrogen-only hormone replacement, inherited high-risk malignancy mutations (primarily Lynch syndrome) and diabetes and hypertension, primarily by their association with obesity (a surrogate marker).

Other types of uterine cancers include adenosquamous carcinoma, mixed Müllerian tumour, papillary serous, clear cell carcinoma and uterine muscle cancers, called sarcomas. These are biologically more aggressive and have a worse prognosis than endometrial adenocarcinoma.

Endometrial cancer

As outline above, the majority of tumours are endometrial adenocarcinoma.

Clinical features The cardinal clinical feature is post-menopausal bleeding and 10% of women with post-menopausal bleeding will have endometrial malignancy, pre-menopausal women who develop endometrial cancer present with menorrhagia and inter-menstrual bleeding.

Endometrial cancer tissue is unstable with a rich blood supply and this is the reason for the abnormal bleeding, which also means that the cancer is also usually identified at an early stage when easily cured by surgery.

Endometrial cancer metastasises locally, directly through the vagina, uterus, fallopian tubes and to the ovaries as well as through lymphatics to regional lymph nodes and finally haematogenously, with predilection for the lungs, liver, bones and brain.

Late diagnoses when the disease has spread beyond the uterus are uncommon; however, women will report symptoms of pelvic masses (from spread to the ovaries) or cough/haemoptysis or pain from lung or bony lesions.

Clinical examination is normal in early disease for the abdomen, lymph nodes and genitalia, speculum examination is performed to exclude other local vaginal causes of bleeding such as polyps or atrophic vaginitis and if the woman is bleeding at the time, this can be seen coming from the cervical os. A bulky fixed uterus, lymphadenopathy, hepatomegaly and bony pain can be found in late disease.

Investigations and diagnosis Investigations are radiologic and diagnosis is histological.

The key diagnostic radiologic investigation is pelvic ultrasound as this will report the thickness of the endometrial stripe and presence of intra-cavity pathology that can also cause bleeding including polyps. Once histological diagnosis is made CT is performed to assess for lymph node spread and distant metastases. This should include the chest, abdomen and pelvis as endometrial cancer spreads locally to regional lymph nodes and haematogenously to the lungs and liver. Women with symptoms of cerebral metastasis should also have a CT of the brain.

Management Management is according to surgical stage and staging for this malignancy is surgico-pathological. This means that women who are fit for surgery and who have no evidence of distant disease on CT are offered a either mid-line abdominal open or laparoscopic hysterectomy with removal of fallopian tubes and ovaries (bilateral salpingo-oophorectomy) as well as pelvic lymph node excision and sampling of peritoneal fluid.

This aim is to cure by removing all cancer, but also gives useful prognostic information of risk of recurrence and guides need for adjuvant therapy.

Tumours are divided into early stage (confined to the uterus) and advanced stage (extra-uterine spread) in terms of further management.

Advanced stage tumours require adjuvant therapy, which may not be curative and early-stage tumours with high-risk features are also offered adjuvant therapy to reduce local recurrence risk which is primarily in the vaginal vault.

High-risk features include:
- Myometrial invasion >50% of depth of myometrium
- Grade 2 or 3 histology (high grade)

- Lymphovascular space or vascular invasion
- Cervical extension of tumour

Adjuvant therapy for early-stage tumours is given as radio-therapy to the vaginal vault via and intra-vaginal applicator called vault brachytherapy. This requires post-radiotherapy care with a long-term vaginal dilator and oestrogen to prevent late vaginal stenosis (see clinical insight box).

> ## Clinical insight
>
> Radiotherapy damages DNA, which impairs the ability of malignant cells to divide as their DNA repair mechanisms are faulty. It also damages normal cells and those that rapidly divide such as the gut are particularly affected. For this reason, radiotherapy generally cannot be applied over most of the abdomen as it causes unacceptably severe early side effects.
>
> Radiotherapy also has late side effects in most tissues including stricture, fibrosis and stenosis formation.

Advanced stage (spread beyond the uterus) tumours are offered adjuvant therapy with radiotherapy to the vault and draining lymph node beds and can also be offered chemotherapy. This is most likely if the distant disease is suspected or known to be outside of the possible field of radiotherapy.

Prognosis Early stage endo-metrial cancer without high-risk features has an 80–90% five-year survival rate. Recurrences are usually within 2 years of primary tumour and occur in the vaginal vault if no prior radiotherapy was given and in para-aortic and pelvic lymph nodes and distantly if prior vault radiotherapy has been given.

Late stage tumours have a 10 to 30 percent five-year survival rate.

Uterine muscle cancers

Uterine muscle cancers occur in previously normal muscle (sarcoma and leiomyosarcoma) tissue, but can also develop in pre-existing fibroids (leiomyosarcoma); this is uncommon at <1% of fibroids.

Clinical features Most uterine muscle cancers present with abnormal vaginal bleeding (menorrhagia, inter-menstrual bleeding or post-menopausal bleeding) or symptoms of mass effect due to enlarged uterus (pressure, abdominal distension, urinary frequency and prolapse). Overall, 85% of women have abnormal bleeding.

Many are diagnosed incidentally after hysterectomy is performed for suspected benign cause including fibroids and menorrhagia. This is because imaging appearances overlap with benign causes and uterine muscle cancers are an uncommon cause of a common presentation. Prior pelvic radiotherapy is a risk factor for uterine sarcoma as 10–20% of sarcomas occur in irradiated women, the remainder are sporadic. Peak incidence is post-menopausal.

Uterine muscle cancers are less common than endometrial cancers at 5% of uterine cancers, (endometrial cancers are 95%) and are biologically more aggressive meaning they metastasise earlier, are diagnosed at more advanced stage and also have worse mortality at equivalent stages to endometrial cancer. Spread occurs locally to adjacent structures as well as haematogenously and less commonly through lymphatics.

Investigations and diagnosis Initial investigations include:
- *Pelvic ultrasound*: To identify focal myometrial pathology and exclude abnormal endometrial thickening
- *Cervical screening test*: To exclude a cervical cause for irregular bleeding
- *Hysteroscopy/Endometrial biopsy*: If submucous component to the pathology, this will establish the histological diagnosis, otherwise this will exclude endometrial hyperplasia and endometrial cancer

If diagnosis is suspected before hysterectomy, which is only the case if rapid growth is detected or quality imaging suggests areas of haemorrhage or necrosis also arrange:
- *Lactate dehydrogenase (LDH)*: Tumour marker, which can be elevated in leiomyosarcoma and, therefore, used for later tracking
- *MRI of the pelvis*: Sensitive for sarcomatous changes in focal myometrial lesions but not specific
- *CT of the chest, abdomen and pelvis*: As part of pre-operating staging as for endometrial cancer above

Clinical insight

Choosing the correct skin incision is very important in surgery. A Pfannenstiel incision (horizontal across the bikini line) allows access to the uterus, has less wound dehiscence and post-operative pain; however, it is considerably smaller than a mid-line incision, gives inferior access to the remainder of the pelvic/abdominal contents and no access to the upper abdomen. A vertical mid-line incision is appropriate when wide surgical exposure or exploration is anticipated (such as trauma or cancer surgery) for this reason.

Management Women with a pre-operative diagnosis of confirmed or suspected uterine muscle cancer are treated in a cancer unit, as this improves oncological outcomes and maximises the chance of complete resection. Standard of care for women with suspected or known uterine muscle cancer is a staging laparotomy, meaning mid-line skin incision, removal of the uterus, cervix, fallopian tubes, ovaries and omentum with pelvic washings and biopsies of any suspicious areas of peritoneum.

Women with known extra-uterine disease can be directed primarily to palliative chemotherapy or radiotherapy, however, if surgically possible and the woman is well enough to tolerate the operation, resection of their uterus and primary tumour will help with symptoms of bleeding and pelvic mass and may be done even though cure is not possible for this reason.

Prognosis

Five-year survival rates are lower than for endometrial cancer at 50% for early stage and 10–20% for advanced stage.

9.6 Ovarian cancer

Ovarian cancer is a significant clinical challenge as symptoms are non-specific and the majority of women are diagnosed at advanced stage and die of their disease. Despite intensive efforts to develop an effective screening test, none exist.

There are several broad subtypes of ovarian cancer: epithelial (comprising serous, clear cell, endometrioid and mucinous), germ cell and sex cord-stromal tumours and metastasis (most commonly breast, upper gastrointestinal and bowel). Up to 85% of ovarian cancers are epithelial, 10% are other subtypes and 5% are metastatic tumours. The subtype is important, as it predicts biologic tumour behaviour, risk of metastasis and optimal treatment modality.

Modern suspicion suggests that the fallopian tube epithelium is responsible for the origin of high-grade serous and low-grade serous tumours and clear cell arises from endometriosis rather than the ovary. This is the reason salpingectomies are offered opportunistically when gynaecological surgery occurs in women who have completed childbearing.

Clinical features

Ovarian cancer is known as a great 'mimic' because most symptoms are easily confused with other common less serious problems. It represents around 2% of all female cancers but 4% of cancer deaths and the lifetime risk is around 1:80 for women who are at 'average' risk without a high-risk mutation. The overall five-year survival rate is 46% with 75% being diagnosed at an advanced stage (stages 3 and 4).

Symptoms include bloating, constipation, diarrhoea, reflux, menstrual pattern change and change in weight and waist circumference.

They are caused by accumulation of malignant ascites, mass effect, bowel dysfunction from tumour caking/coating and constitutional symptoms and loss of weight from metabolic drain of the cancer. The pelvic cavity does not have somatic (precise, detailed, like the skin and body surface) innervation and can accommodate a pregnancy to the end of the first trimester without much in the way of external change; it is unsurprising that subtle early symptoms are misattributed and a cancer can be both large and widespread before detection.

Epithelial ovarian cancer spreads by direct extension around the ovaries, fallopian tubes, uterus and more generally around the abdominal cavity, progressively coating the bowel and omentum in tumour deposit. Distant metastases are uncommon and most women die because of direct effects on bowel function (obstruction) or due to tumour-related VTE.

Clear cell and high-grade serous are more aggressive with earlier metastasis and poorer prognosis than other subtypes.

Non-epithelial cancers (germ cell and sex cord-stromal tumours) Germ cell and sex cord-stromal tumours also have symptoms of oestrogen or androgen output including heavy periods, acne and excessive hair grown in a male pattern (beard area and chest). Germ cell tumours metastasise to other sites including lymph nodes, lungs, liver and brain and have peak incidence in children. All other types are most common in post-menopausal women.

Investigations and diagnosis

Investigations Investigations are haematological and radiological. They include, in order, a vaginal pelvic US scan to identify the presence of an ovarian cyst and blood test for ovarian tumour marker levels.

The routine tumour marker is cancer antigen 125 (CA 125) and depending on clinical suspicion can also include LDH (dysgerminoma – a germ cell tumour), CA 19-9 (mucinous tumours and dermoid cysts), alpha-fetoprotein (AFP) (yolk sac – a germ cell tumour and bowel cancer), CA 15-3 (breast cancer), inhibin (granulosa tumours) and oestrogen/testosterone (sex cord-stromal tumours).

> ## Clinical insight
>
> Vaginal transducers perform significantly better at identifying pelvic pathology for two key reasons; they are physically very close to the uterus and ovary to use a high frequency waveform which gives fine image resolution.
>
> This is because ultrasound ability to travel through tissue is inversely related to wavelength and when an abdominal transducer is used, the much greater distance to the pelvis requires a lower frequency transducer with significant loss of image quality.

The US scan will also identify increased endometrial thickness if present (from tumour hormonal output) as well as signs the cyst is malignant. These include rapid growth from a prior scan, combination of cystic and solid areas, internal papillary projections, low resistance Doppler flow and presence of ascites, bilateral ovarian pathology and metastases in the pouch of Douglas.

In cases where malignancy is diagnosed (e.g. post-oophorectomy or cystectomy with cancer in the specimen) or very likely (evidence of bilateral complex cysts with ascites), a CT scan of the chest abdomen and pelvis is also performed to assess for degree of local and distant metastases.

Diagnosis Diagnosis is histological or cytological; meaning is made examining either malignant fluid or tissue in the laboratory.

The majority of cases are strongly suspected due to investigations above with or without the addition of a risk of malignancy index (RMI) calculation and are operated on in a cancer unit and final diagnosis is then made.

Some cases are diagnosed incidentally when a cystectomy or oophorectomy is performed for presumed benign pathology and cancer is identified histologically.

A minority of cases are diagnosed when either ascites or pleural effusion is drained and malignant ovarian cells are identified in the fluid without having had a prior surgical histological diagnosis.

Women who have an incidental unexpected histological diagnosis will usually need further surgery to attempt cure them of their cancer and women who have a cytological diagnosis on

Good practice point

It is tempting to perform blood tumour marker tests in women with vague symptoms, but this should be avoided.

'Blind' tumour marker tests are poor practice, as nearly all tumour markers are neither very specific for malignancy nor sensitive enough to perform acceptably as a diagnostic test.

This is because many non-cancer diagnoses can cause elevation such as endometriosis. In the cause of ovarian cancer they also particularly lack sensitivity as CA 125 is normal in 50% of stage one tumours.

In other words, the test will not detect a tumour before ultrasound and only adds diagnostic utility, if a suspicious cyst is present. Monitoring of known cancer for recurrence is different and this is an acceptable use of the blood test alone as a raise after decline is suspicious for recurrence.

Good practice point

Risk of malignancy index, or RMI, is a simple calculator that aids decision-making on suitable site and mode of surgery for ovarian cysts. It is generated by multiplying menopausal score (1 for pre and 3 for post) by CA 125 number by ultrasound score (1 for no suspicious features, 2 for one suspicious feature and 3 for ≥two suspicious features; suspicious features are bilaterality, multi-loculated, solid/cystic, ascites and metastases).

Scores >200 are suspicious for malignancy and should be managed in a cancer unit.

malignant ascites and pleural effusion are usually too advanced to benefit from routine surgical excision. Both should be urgently referral to a gynaecological cancer unit.

Management

Management of ovarian cancer is primarily surgical with curative intent, meaning with intention to resect all disease.

There is also a significant role for additional treatment with chemotherapy either before surgery (neo-adjuvant) in order to increase resectability or after surgery (adjuvant) to reduce risk of recurrence or treat known metastases and prolong survival.

Early-stage tumours Early-stage tumours are treated by staging laparotomy. This entails a mid-line skin incision (for wide access to the abdomen including upper abdomen), peritoneal washings, removal of uterus, fallopian tubes, ovaries and omentum and palpation of the liver and diaphragms for metastatic disease in this location. Any suspected metastases are also removed, if in a resectable location, which can also require bowel resection.

Diet is introduced slowly post-operatively as there is a high ileus risk from bowel handling/surgery and extended VTE prophylaxis for 4–6 weeks is also given as cancer increases the change of a VTE event. Women also benefit from early review with a physiotherapist for mobility and chest infection preventative strategies and proton pump inhibitor therapy to reduce the incidence of stress ulceration. Pre-menopausal women are given oestrogen alone menopausal hormone therapy.

Most women will subsequently receive adjuvant chemotherapy and all are followed-up clinically and biochemically with CA 125 (if elevated pre-operatively) and with imaging, if symptoms, signs or abnormal CA 125 level at regular intervals for 5–10 years in a cancer unit to detect recurrence.

Advanced stage tumour Advanced stage tumour care is individualised. Some women are suitable for surgery to debulk their disease to minimal residual to prolong survival, enhance chemotherapy response and reduce symptoms of advanced ovarian cancer (ascites, pain from pelvic mass, ileus and bowel obstruction).

Other women are offered palliative chemotherapy to prolong survival.

Other cares are directed to relieving symptoms and improving quality of life.

Germ cell tumours These are managed differently; germ cell tumours occur in young women and are extremely chemosensitive, so surgery is usually fertility sparing (removal of the affected ovary) with chemotherapy and carries a good prognosis.

Prognosis

Overall five-year survival rates are 70–90% for early tumours and 15–59% for advanced disease. Women who die of ovarian cancer generally do as a consequence of malignant bowel obstruction or VTE.

Index

Note: Page numbers in **bold** or *italic* refer to tables or figures respectively.